AF326981

The American Health Care System—Betrayed by Greed

The American Health Care System—Betrayed by Greed

Esmond H. Coleman

VANTAGE PRESS
New York

FIRST EDITION

All rights reserved, including the right of
reproduction in whole or in part in any form.

Copyright © 1993 by Esmond H. Coleman

Published by Vantage Press, Inc.
516 West 34th Street, New York, New York 10001

Manufactured in the United States of America
ISBN: 0-533-10494-7

Library of Congress Catalog Card No.: 92-94296

0 9 8 7 6 5 4 3 2 1

Contents

Foreword
by Philip R. Lee, M.D.

Today the American health care system is undergoing a vast change. Because of the rapid and continuous escalation of costs, a new mandate is emerging that challenges the traditional values that have formed the underpinnings of our health care system for generations.

In response to rapidly rising costs, the three major payers—the federal government, state governments, and employers—have developed a variety of strategies to slow the rate of increase of health care costs. Each sector, public and private, has tried to limit its costs and shift the burden to the other or to the consumer. In an effort to increase competition, third parties have increased cost-sharing by beneficiaries, promoted health maintenance organizations, emphasized utilization review and managed care, and used a variety of measures to regulate hospitals and physicians. These strategies have had limited success in containing cost increases and, unfortunately, have had serious consequences for many Americans in terms of access to affordable health care.

The concept that all citizens are entitled to adequate health care, which emerged with the enactment of Medicare and Medicaid in 1965, is rapidly being replaced by the concept that the market is the arbiter of access. Many of those responsible for health care financing now maintain that limited available finances must be rationed in some fashion. However disguised that change, the result is different levels of care—from excellent to adequate, from bad to nonexistent—depending on wealth, social class, race, age, employment status, disease, and place of residence. An estimated 37 million Americans are now uninsured and depend on charity or local governments to provide care when they are in need.

Issues related to health care access, costs, and financing are the subject of a growing number of studies reported in thousands of articles in newspapers, magazines, and in professional journals, books, television programs, government committee hearings, and professional forums across the country. Unfortunately, the quality, accuracy, and clarity of the information available to the interested parties vary considerably. Some of the studies have focused on small segments of the problem. These include the exposure of abuses by one or more nursing homes or hospitals, trials of physicians charged with Medicaid fraud, pharmaceutical companies producing faulty and/or overpriced drugs, and other tales of fraud and abuse.

Other studies have compared the advantages and disadvantages of Medicare and Medicaid, or have exhaustively analyzed the different types of hospitals and the effect on them of various types of medical insurance. Another class of research studies has analyzed health statistics relating to infant mortality, life expectancy, and the amount spent on health care as a percentage of gross national product.

While some of the results of the work have been useful to limited audiences, other results have been of little practical value. Even some of the books and articles written by physicians put more emphasis on technical matters, specific diseases, and medical theories than on issues of concern to the public.

The common factor in the studies, government pronouncements, and the popular press is a lack of concern for or focus on the most important element of all—the consumer. For example, infant mortality rates, life expectancy, days of hospital stay in the event of acute illness, and other similar measures are normally expressed as national averages. While that level of detail may be appropriate for federal policymakers, it is not the focus for consumers who are interested in their community clinic, local hospital, or health department. Much more meaningful, and what people want to know, is information that applies directly to specific consumer groups such as the affluent, poor, black, white, Hispanic, aged, indigent, resident of an inner city or of a rural town, or any combination of these groups.

The great value of this book, *The American Health Care System—Betrayed by Greed*, is that it is written from the consumer's point of view, in language that everyone can understand. Nowhere in it are there broad generalizations or grand patriotic slogans. Rather, this is a measured book that considers both the benefits and inadequacies of health care, as well as the fragmentation of financing and consequent inequalities of care. It is not, like some other books on the subject, a filtered listing of the dramatic cases of fraud and abuse. *The American Health Care System—Betrayed by Greed* frequently uses actual case studies to present clearly what is happening at the everyday consumer level of health care.

Just as important as its objective treatment of the subject, however, is this book's forthright and bold demonstration of what we, the citizens of the richest country in the world, can do to stop trying to fix the health care system with a patchwork of half-remedies, and move on to the essential task of instituting a comprehensive and effective cure.

—Philip R. Lee, M.D.
Professor of Social Medicine
University of California, San Francisco

Preface

Many books and articles have been written on one or more aspects of our health care system; some have been very informative and have exposed atrocious examples of inadequacy, waste, fraud, and abuse. This book, however, is different for several reasons; I shall mention two of them here. In the first place, it is far more comprehensive, assessing all of the actors in the rapidly developing tragedy. In the second place, it has been written from a fiscal point of view. A description of my qualifications in this area is in order here.

Health Care Experience

For many years I was the certified public accountant (CPA) for a large home health agency and a hospice program on the West Coast of the United States. These two types of agencies will be described in detail in the chapters that follow. Acting as a CPA and auditor, I had to interpret the Medicare and Medicaid laws and regulations promulgated by the federal government in 1965 and thereafter. As I shall make clear, this was not a routine task; it involved the education of government personnel, the staff of the fiscal intermediaries appointed by the government to reimburse providers of Medicare and Medicaid services, and CPAs selected by the government to audit the costs claimed by the providers. In a number of cases, the government personnel and their appointees were poorly trained and did not understand what they were doing. In November 1986, when the San Francisco Home Health Service (SFHHS) was merged into one of San Francisco's major hospitals, Hadley Dale Hall, the executive director of the SFHHS, and Michael A. Roosevelt, executive director of the Hospice of San Francisco, evaluated my 25 years of service as follows:

> Through his clear exposition, Medicare came to understand the functions of the homemaker/home health aide, and how they fit into Medicare's complex accounting. The accuracy of his facts and figures were always evident—in spite of a constant changing cadre of government employees who nearly always started

with different assumptions and incorrect facts.

Esmond H. Coleman has been responsible for accurate accounting for millions of dollars which served the ill, the dying and the poor. The people of San Francisco are grateful and thankful.

When the AIDS epidemic was identified in 1981, I became conversant with the governmental inadequacy and refusal to take the problem seriously. That will be amplified later.

In 1972, the first public interest organization of certified public accountants in the United States opened its doors in San Francisco, California.[1] It was named Accountants for the Public Interest (API). I was one of its founders and its first president. The main purpose of API was to provide accounting consultation to nonprofit organizations and groups of people who were engaged in public interest actions or investigations. These consultations provided accounting interpretation and analysis which the organizations and groups could not pay for because of their limited finances.

Although the few organizers of API were optimistic about the future, we were not prepared for the rapid growth we experienced. The reason for the interest was that the student unrest during the 1960s involved not only the political and free speech issues but the whole question of relevance of learning. Some students studying accounting and young CPAs felt that their professional skills should be used not only to earn a handsome living but should also be utilized to help solve social problems. It is sad to observe that, to a large extent, during the 1980s and in the 1990s social problems do not seem particularly important to CPAs. In any case, in the 1970s API flourished not only in San Francisco, but we were able to open offices in Portland (Oregon), Los Angeles, Philadelphia, Washington, D.C., New York, Newark, Chicago, Providence, Boston, Helena (Montana), Miami, Denver, and Austin.

Foundations provided the necessary funds (in San Francisco) to maintain an office and pay for a skeleton office force; the CPAs volunteered their services and API charged no fees. The work consisted of analytical studies designed to enable the applicants to understand the pertinent issues facing them, and to use the studies and API personnel to frame their arguments. API maintained a nonadvocacy stance, adhered strictly to professional standards, but performed no audits.

Prior to the formation of API, which in a sense was the counterpart of the public interest law firm, CPA societies and CPAs individually had rendered some assistance on a pro bono basis to the public, assisting small businesses, taxpayers who needed help they could not afford, etc., but this was the first time that a CPA organization, on a planned basis, made its services available to needy groups. Many issues were addressed by API. I am listing a few here to illustrate the scope of our vision:

- An investigation of the estimated cost for the care of dependent, abused, and neglected children in San Francisco. The purpose of this investigation was to segregate the costs of caring for these children, as contrasted with delinquent children, all of whom were housed in the Youth Guidance Center and several ancillary facilities. The ultimate purpose was to determine whether a better, more economical method could be devised to care for the dependent, abused and neglected group.
- A study of the fiscal problems relating to the proposed expansion of the San Francisco Airport (1973 case).
- A study of the operation of a community college.
- An analysis of the relative fiscal advantages of maintaining an open space area in an undeveloped area as opposed to developing housing, etc.
- The Hill-Burton case in New Orleans (covered later in this book).
- A study of San Francisco nursing homes (covered later in this book).
- A study of hospital management firms (covered later in this book).

I have listed a few of the cases handled by API, and there were many more. Because I had many years of experience in the health field, I became the leader of "The Health Group" within API. In that capacity, by performing extensive research and exacting analyses, I learned the ingenious and at times ludicrous techniques devised by the government, health care providers and their associates to evade their legal and ethical responsibilities.

Back to World War II

To some, the spectacle of chaos in governmental program planning might have been an amazing experience, but in my case, it was more a case of déjà vu, because during World War II, as a lieutenant in the Corps of Engineers, I was assigned to participate in the enforcement of the Renegotiation Act, a law enacted with the express purpose of preventing the flagrant profiteering that had occurred during World War I. The plan was to audit business enterprises and recover "excessive profits" earned by them for services and supplies used in the war effort. Obviously, to recover "excessive profits" it would have been helpful to know what that term meant. This is how Title VII, Renegotiation of War Contracts (a public law enacted during the 78th Congress of the U.S.A., 1944) defined it:

> The term "excessive profits" means the profits derived from contracts with the Department and subcontracts, which is determined in accordance with this section to be excessive. In determining excessive profits there shall be taken into consideration the following factors:
> (i) efficiency of contractors, with particular regard to attainment of quantity production, reduction of costs . . . economy . . . ;
> (ii) reasonableness of costs and profits, with particular regard to volume . . . prewar earnings, and comparison of prewar earnings, and comparison of war and peacetime products;
> (iii) amount and source of public and private capital employed and net worth;

In addition, other factors were included related to risks involved, contribution to the war effort, cooperation with the government and other contributors providing technical assistance, complexity of the manufacturing techniques, consideration of public interest and equitable dealing, and other regulations to be issued from time to time.

The only thing not mentioned by the Act was where we who were responsible for determining "excessive profits" could purchase a crystal ball.

In order to understand the problem, consider the case of a hardware store in a small town. Before the war it was fairly profitable, with a 10% net profit of $15,000 on annual sales of $150,000. During the war, it secured a contract to fabricate landing barges for the navy. Its sales increased to $1,500,000, with a net profit of 12%, or $180,000. In this case, what constitutes a fair profit? $30,000? $50,000? $100,000? 7%? 9%? 12%? Nobody really knew the answer, so that in each industry, certain percentages were arrived at, and when you encountered a particular type of industry, you learned to examine previous cases and attempted to conform. Those who were doing the work, like myself with a small army salary, were warned never to say to the nouveau riche entrepreneurs, "What about the lowly private in the army earning a pittance?" As a matter of fact, in one case, when I informed a contractor that I was recommending a substantial refund of profits, he responded, "But I won't be able to restock my deer farm!"

But these matters do not really get to the core problem, which is "What is war work?" because unless the project is war work, renegotiation or refund is not applicable. On the face of it, it sounds simple, but is it? If you sell a yacht to a private citizen it is not war work; if you sell a landing barge to the navy, it is. The same principle applies to other products, such as furniture, automobile equipment, steel shelves, food, etc., but even that is too simplistic a formulation. Returning to the Renegotiation Act, we find that the recovery of "excessive profits" does not apply to:

> Any contract or subcontract for the product of a mine, oil or gas well, or other mineral or natural product, or timber, which has not been processed, or treated beyond the first form or state suitable for industrial use.

So—profits earned on pig iron were not renegotiable, on steel yes, on most chemicals no, on copper no. What was the result of this provision? The giant industries at the time, Anaconda Copper, DuPont Industries, big steel, little steel, etc., were exempt from renegotiation.

The largest case I personally audited (together with an assistant) was a large steel company in Ohio. I kept asking for more and more books, ledgers, schedules, etc., until I was firmly convinced that the corporation was maintaining two sets of books, one for tax purposes and one for renegotiation purposes. The latter set proved that most of the profit of the business was earned on the production from iron ore to pig iron, and very little from pig iron to steel; hence the company claimed a clearance, or exemption from returning excessive profits to the government. When I reported my findings to my superiors, they had me travel to other areas, such as New York and Chicago, to ascertain how other steel companies had fared in their renegotiation audits. I learned that all of them had received clearances. I was then overruled by my superiors on my audit. The firm in Ohio also was granted a clearance.

All of the preceding emphasizes that whenever we deal with laws and regulations, whether in the health care field or other fields, we must look at what the various actors do, and what they do not do, what the laws say and what they do not say, how they are interpreted or misinterpreted, how they are enforced or not enforced. What is true of laws and regulations is also true of other aspects of our health care system. My experience and training have provided me with the investigative tools to determine whether the money and effort to provide an effective system have succeeded or failed—and why.

To ensure medical authenticity, three eminent physicians have participated in the preparation and review of this book.

Dr. Philip R. Lee was the assistant secretary for health and scientific affairs of the Federal Department of Health, Education and Welfare from 1965 to 1969 under President Carter. He is also the past chancellor of the University of California Medical School in San Francisco. He is now a professor of social medicine at the University's School of Medicine. Perhaps most pertinent to this book, he has served as the chairman of the Physician Payment Review Commission established by the United States Congress. Dr. Lee has written the foreword to this book and has acted as an advisor on the scope of information.

Dr. Benson Roe is a world-renowned cardiologist who is a past president of the California Academy of Medicine. He is also a professor of surgery and former chief of cardio-thoracic surgery at the University of California, San Francisco. His awards and other accomplishments fill several pages of his curriculum vitae. Now in the process of retiring after a long, distinguished, and successful practice, he provides information seen through the eyes of a physician who has lived intimately with the changes in American medicine. He brings not only his professional standing to this book, but a belief in the future of American medicine as a national right.

Dr. Thomas Bodenheimer is an assistant professor at the California School of Medicine and has served as a Peace Corps physician in Costa Rica. He has been on the National Committee for Human Rights, the governing board of the American Public Health Association, and the National Steering Committee of Physicians for a National Health Program. He was on a 30-member writing committee that helped write a landmark article entitled "A National Health Program for the United States: A Physician's Proposal." Published in the *New England Journal of Medicine,* the article was endorsed by 412 other physicians representing virtually every state and medical specialty. The article is a clear call for a national system of health care and a return to the more altruistic roots of patient care. Dr. Bodenheimer has written the introduction and concluding chapter of this book and in so doing has laid out the details of a comprehensive plan for a national health care system in the United States.

After describing the parlous state of our health care system, this book then proceeds to state what we can do to remedy it. I am referring to a national health care system. The United States is the only developed country in the world other than South Africa that does not have one. But I am not talking about a sudden utopia. I am advocating a reasonable process of change. It should embrace the study of health care systems in other countries, comparing our system with theirs, selecting what is best in each, antagonizing as few people and institutions as possible, and designing a system with health care for all at a cost we can afford. It should also include a comprehensive component of preventive medicine. A recent tri-nation poll[2] makes it abundantly clear that an overwhelming majority of the American people prefer the Canadian national health care system to our present American system.

Why should they not? As it stands now, unless you are a very healthy millionaire, it is not safe to be alive in the United States.

Acknowledgments

This book would never have seen the light of day had it not been for the amazing patience, support, and masochism of my relatives, friends, and associates. My wife, Julia (aka Judy), daughter, Diana, son, Paul, sister Beatrice, brother-in-law Morris, have listened for a decade to my obsessive monologues on the subject of the deficiencies of American health care. For a decade, Julia and Paul have not only listened, they have typed, proofread, and contributed significantly to the content of the book.

Hadley Dale Hall, former executive director of the San Francisco Home Health Service, has taught me much of what I know of our health system and has carefully reviewed the manuscript in detail.

Many members of Accountants for the Public Interest (API) have contributed to my knowledge; a number of them are mentioned in the text. I am grateful to Morton Levy, CPA, for initially defining the concept of API, and to Virginia Hubbell for helping develop it.

Marilyn Rose, Andreas Schneider, and Gordon Bonnyman, all lawyers of public interest law firms, were most valuable to me.

A number of health care experts were generous enough to review portions of the manuscript and make valuable suggestions. I am referring to Alan Abel (Kaiser), Stephen L. Becker, M.D. (University of California), Robert J. Erickson, chief counsel (Kaiser), Val J. Halamandaris, president (National Association for Home Care), Robert H. Lucas, C.E.O. (San Francisco Home Care), Ruth Roemer, adjunct professor of public health (U.C.L.A.), Allan Rosenfeld, M.D., dean of School of Public Health (Columbia University), and William B. Shekter, M.D., Department of Ophthalmology (Kaiser).

Finally, I must mention Dave Myers, a writer who has consistently encouraged my efforts, and Alice Kleeman, who with her trusty computer has persistently enabled me to keep my head above water.

Introduction
by Thomas S. Bodenheimer, M.D.

One can say many negative things about health care in America, Those minuses are not the whole story. Our nation has thousands of fine physicians, nurses, pharmacists, and other health care–givers who compassionately provide a high quality of care to everyone. But at the same time, the health system is a huge conveyor belt transporting billions of dollars from working Americans to wealthy specialty physicians, overpaid administrators, and rich investors in the drug and insurance industries. This is the face of the health system that will be discussed in this book, because this is what urgently needs reform.

"The health care economy of the United States is a paradox of excess and deprivation."[1] In our nation, we have hospitals with 60% of their beds empty turning away patients because they have no insurance. That image is the essence of our health system.

Deprivation

- Timmy Dawkins, son of a small town schoolteacher, developed cancer; the following year the insurance company hiked premiums to all the school's employees by 200%, and 20 other companies refused to insure the school at all.
- Buzz Gammel, owner of a small business, developed a brain tumor; a few months later his insurance announced a rate increase from $1,352 to $10,068 per month, which Mr. Gammel was unable to afford.
- Dean Meyer, former director of the California Insurance Brokers Association, developed coronary artery disease; the only insurance he can obtain has a preexisting illness clause, denying benefits for any costs associated with heart disease.
- In 1989, New York Life Insurance cancelled five group plans, leaving 120,000 individuals without coverage. One of those was James Snyder, a lawyer who had just contracted

leukemia. He was unable to obtain new coverage.
* Ronald Katz, an architect, had two insurance policies cancelled—United of Omaha and Blue Cross—after he contracted AIDS.
* An uninsured janitor in his 30s with rheumatic heart disease was admitted to a coronary care unit, where his bill came to $26,000. To pay the bill he was forced to sell his car, which he used to travel to work. As a result he lost his job and was forced onto welfare.
* When a fifty-nine-year-old woman retired from her job as a bookkeeper, she converted her group insurance to an individual policy. After three years she missed one monthly insurance payment, at which time her insurance was cancelled. When she reapplied for coverage, she was rejected due to high blood pressure.
* A thirty-five-year-old employed black man came to a private hospital emergency room with fever and cough—he had delayed treatment due to lack of health insurance. He was found to have acute leukemia, potentially curable with chemotherapy. Due to treatment delay, the illness was too far advanced and after several months of heroic measures, he died.
* A fifty-eight-year-old Hispanic clerical worker had restrictive lung disease from a spine deformity. She depended on a home Intermittent Positive Pressure (IPPB) machine to assist her breathing. She was finally forced to resign from her job, lost her insurance, and could not afford to rent the IPPB machine. The medical supply company came and took the machine away.
* A man whose Medicaid benefits were terminated died of a treatable perforated ulcer because he delayed seeking care for 10 days. An uninsured cardiac patient died of a presumed myocardial infarction after running out of cardiac medications that he could not afford to buy. A hypertensive patient without health insurance died of a stroke after becoming unable to afford her blood pressure medications.
* Two neurosurgeons at a private hospital refused to see a young uninsured man who was going into a coma after a severe beating in the head. The patient died shortly after being transferred to a county hospital.[2]

Excess

- Secretary of Health and Human Services, Dr. Louis Sullivan, estimates that as much as 25% of all medical procedures performed may be inappropriate or unnecessary.
- "A third if not more than half of what we do now is of no benefit or of so marginal a benefit that I think we could agree in society that insurance should not pay for it."
- Carotid endarterectomy (surgery unclogging the arteries flowing to the brain) was found to be inappropriately performed in 32% of the cases studied.
- Only 56% of 386 coronary bypass operations performed in three randomly chosen California hospitals were clearly justified. 30% were equivocal and 14% were found to be inappropriate.
- 20% of cardiac pacemaker implants are not necessary and an additional 36% are ambiguous.
- At least a quarter of the 1.7 million cataract surgeries performed on Americans each year are unnecessary.
- A Rand Corporation study of Medicare patients found that 40% of their medications are unnecessary and 15% of seniors' hospitalizations result from reactions to inappropriate medications.[3]

Administrative waste consumes 20% to 25% of the nation's entire health expenditures.[4]

Overall, according to Dr. Robert Brook, Professor at UCLA, "almost every study that has seriously looked for overuse has discovered it, and virtually every time at least double-digit overuse has been found. If one could extrapolate from the available literature, then perhaps one-fourth of hospital days, one-fourth of procedures, and two-fifths of medications could be done without."[5]

The Crossroads

In 1950, the United States came to a health care crossroads. The Wagner-Murray-Dingell bill for national health insurance, first introduced into the U.S. Congress in 1943, had been endorsed by President Harry Truman in 1945—the first and last time an American president supported national health insurance. After Truman's election victory of 1948, the bill had a chance; it would have placed the entire population under a single publicly financed health insurance system. The American Medical Association waged an all-out campaign against Wagner-Murray-Dingell in 1949. The bill died, and the nation's best chance at national health insurance died with it.

The alternative to national health insurance was consummated in 1965 with the passage of Medicare and Medicaid. These programs provided government health insurance to the elderly and some of the poor, allowing the private insurance industry to cover middle- and upper-income people. This retreat from national health insurance set up a dual system of health care: private insurance for the healthier segments of the population and public insurance for older, sicker, and poorer people. The division of the population between public and private is the root cause of the paradox of excess and deprivation. Those people who are well insured (which includes the higher-income elderly who generally have both Medicare and private insurance) may receive too much care because their care earns income for the providers and suppliers of health care. Those who are poor or chronically disabled (needing long-term care) suffer inadequate care because their Medicaid card pays providers too little or because they have no card at all and remain uninsured.

The rule governing American health care is: if you walk into the doctor's office or the hospital admitting office with a card (Medicare, private insurance) that offers good reimbursement to the doctor and the hospital, you are welcomed, and in fact, subject to overtreatment. Excess. If you walk into a doctor's office or hospital with a Medicaid card, or no card at all, or into a nursing home where Medicare and private insurance rarely guarantee reimbursement, then you are treated as a second-class citizen and are subject to undertreatment. Deprivation. The nation's chance to place everyone under one single equal system was lost in 1950, and is only now back on the public agenda.

Who Pays for Health Care in America?

CATEGORY	POPULATION (millions)	%
Employer-sponsored private insurance, under age sixty-five	145	58
Individual private insurance, under age sixty-five	21	8
Medicare	33	13
Total with desirable health coverage	199	79
No insurance coverage	32	13
Medicaid	20	8
Total	251	100

From the point of view of health care providers, the most "desirable" patients measured in terms of reimbursement rates are those with private health insurance or Medicare. Thus, 199 million people have "desirable" health coverage. Subtracting those ten million severely disabled people whose coverage rarely pays for needed long-term care, 189 million or about 75% of the population can be considered "desirable," and at risk for excessive care. The other 25% (the uninsured, Medicaid recipients, and those needing long-term care) can be thought of as "undesirable" patients and at risk for insufficient health care.

Looking at payment for health care according to dollars rather than population, about 27% of health care dollars are paid by employer-sponsored private health insurance, 5% by individual health insurance, 21% out-of-pocket, 5% by philanthropy and other private funds, and 42% by government programs (chiefly Medicare and Medicaid).[6] Who really pays these dollars? In fact, for the 53% coming from private insurance and out-of-pocket payments, lower-income families pay a greater proportion of their income than higher-income families, thereby making these payments unfairly regressive.

It is easy to see why out-of-pocket payments are regressive. If you pay the doctor $500 and your income is $5000, you have paid 10% of income. But if your income is $50,000, the $500 represents only 1% of your income. What makes the situation even worse is that sicker people—who need more care—tend to have lower incomes, so that if you earn $5000, you probably pay the doctor $700, which is 14% of your income, whereas the healthier person earning $50,000 rarely seeks care and pays only $250, which is 0.5% of income. Individual insurance is similarly regressive. Your insurance premium may be $500, 10% of your income if you earn $5000, but 1% if you earn $50,000. And sicker people, who tend to have lower incomes, are generally charged higher premiums, thereby aggravating the inequities.

Employer-sponsored health insurance, though a bit more complicated, operates under the same principle. Whereas it appears that employers pay most of the premium costs, in fact, economists have analyzed that over the long run, these costs are actually deducted from wages and salaries. Thus, employees earning $5000 are spending 10% of their wage on a $500 insurance premium; employees making $50,000 spend only 1%.

The government programs are financed somewhat more fairly, with health care payments (in taxes and social security contributions) rising as income rises. But taking all health care expenses—premiums, taxes, and out-of-pocket payments—families with the lowest 10% of incomes pay about 20% of their income for health care, while the highest 10% of income earners pay only 8.4% of their incomes for health care.[7] It should be evident that health care in America is financed in a highly inequitable fashion.

Who Benefits from American Health Expenditures?

Now that we know where the money comes from, where does it go? Every dollar going into the health system looks like costs to consumers, but looks like income or profits for providers, suppliers, and insurers of health care. Billions of dollars are spent to pay the hardworking physicians, nurses, hospital maintenance and dietary workers, and millions of others who make the health system run day after day. But too many billions are spent to enrich a small number of overpaid professionals and investors. Let us first look at the general destinations of health care dollars, and then explore behind the scenes to uncover instances of overpayment, profit and waste—expenditures that perhaps could be reduced.

Of the $540 billion spent on health care in 1988, 39% went to hospital care, 19% to physician services, 8% to nursing homes, 22% to other personal health care (including dental, home health care, medications, and medical equipment) and 12% to other categories such as administration, research, and construction. Let us analyze some of these expenditures in a more critical light.

A considerable proportion of the 39% going for hospital expenditures is questionable in terms of medical appropriateness. According to Professor Robert Brook, 25% of hospital days are unnecessary.[8] In addition, about 40% of hospital beds in the U.S. are empty on any given day, with an empty bed costing about two-thirds of a full bed. If we could eliminate half the empty beds and all of the unneeded hospital days, we could save $80 billion each year.

Hidden within the 19% going to physicians are huge differences in the incomes of different specialties. The average primary physician's income in 1990 was about $100,000. The average specialist's income was about $161,000, with some specialists earning upwards of $500,000. Let us assume that specialists deserve an average income of $135,000, with the excess above that level considered to be overpayment. Given that the U.S. enjoys about 237,000 specialists, the excess income of specialists totals about $6 billion per year. Eliminating the professional cost of the 25% of procedures (surgical and diagnostic) that are inappropriately performed[9] would save an additional $15 billion.

The pharmaceutical industry is one of the most lucrative sectors of the American economy, earning profits close to twice those of the average manufacturing corporation. If we assume one-half of the $6 billion in drug industry profits to be excessive, we could save $3 billion per year. In addition, two-fifths of medications are probably unnecessarily prescribed; were these unneeded prescriptions to be eliminated, we could save another $16 billion.[10]

For the insurance industry, profits on health care are difficult to determine because they are mixed in with profits from other insurance products such as life insurance. On the other hand, the administrative costs of the private health insurance industry come to 12%, about four times the 3% administrative costs of government health insurance programs such as Medicare and Medicaid. Reducing insurance industry administrative costs to the 3% figure for government programs could save $8 billion per year.

Adding up this list of excess spending, the United States could save $138 billion by reducing unnecessary care and administrative waste. This is most certainly a conservative figure; some authors have estimated a potential savings of $70–80 billion in administrative waste and $160–270 billion in medical excess.[11]

Overcoming Excess and Deprivation

We have shown that the American health system suffers from both excess and deprivation: excess for the 75% who are well insured, deprivation for the 25% who are poorly insured or uninsured. The excess is costly in terms of dollars; the deprivation is costly in terms of lives.

In order to overcome the paradox of excess and deprivation, we must eliminate the dual system of care and cover all Americans under a single national health insurance plan. A unitary public insurance system can 1) treat everyone equally and thereby eliminate deprivation, and 2) apply firm cost controls to reduce administrative and medical waste and thereby cut down on excess.

If we want to change the health system, we cannot count on the providers or insurers of care to do it for us. Remember, every dollar we spend on health care is a dollar in the pocket of someone working in the health system. As we noted above, most of those dollars are well earned, by nurses, pharmacists, hospital workers, community mental health providers, and decent, hardworking physicians. But we cannot forget that billions of those dollars help to enrich wealthy specialists, drug company and insurance company executives, who do not want to give up those extra dollars. The AMA, the Health Insurance Association of America, the pharmaceutical companies—these and other groups will not act in the interest of the majority of the American people. It will take health care consumers and dedicated, unselfish health care workers to eliminate the excesses and the deprivations of the U.S. health care system.

The American Health Care System—Betrayed by Greed

such as Medicare, Medicaid, or insurance companies. Those costs are not reflected on the books or financial statements of the hospital.

A study performed in the 1970s by API (an organization discussed in the preface) disclosed that about one-half of the cost of a hip replacement operation in a large urban hospital was to be found in hospital records. The other half comprised bills rendered directly by surgeons and anesthesiologists to patients and third party payers. This fact is never disclosed to the public by physicians, hospitals, or certified public accountants.

The increase in the number of hospitals, once they became institutions where the sick could be cured, was very dramatic. This was facilitated by improved medical technology, sanitation, transportation, and the amelioration of the overall economy attendant upon the industrial revolution and the upgraded education, social and financial status of physicians. The number of hospitals in the United States, in 1987, for example, was as follows:[4]

Nongovernmental Nonprofit	3,338
Nongovernmental for Profit	834
State and Local Government	1,556
Long-term	133
Federal	342
Miscellaneous	638
Total	6,841

At this point, however, I shall return to a somewhat earlier period in American history.

The Great Depression, which followed the stock market crash of 1929, caused widespread unemployment and ushered in a period of trade union organization and desperate, militant action on the part of the working class in the United States. Social Security and unemployment insurance were established by law. People demanded comprehensive medical care, not as a privilege for the deserving poor, but as a right for all. Public opinion polls demonstrated the overwhelming support for such a program.

The government, under the leadership of President Franklin Roosevelt, dragged its feet and the pressure petered out. World War II in the early 1940s focused the attention of the United States on other matters, but immediately after the War, the United States was turning back to domestic concerns. One of the gravest problems was the poor state of health of vast numbers of Americans, attributable in large part to the shortage of medical facilities, the deplorable condition of those in existence, and the lack of access to those facilities by people in the lower income brackets. That had been attested to by the large number of draftees judged unfit for military service for health reasons. A large segment of the American population was demanding some form of national health insurance.

Shortly before he died, President Roosevelt seemed convinced that health insurance should be established, and in 1945, his successor, Harry Truman, called on Congress to pass a national program to assure adequate medical care. The public was very supportive of this view.[5]

The American Medical Association (AMA) saw things somewhat differently. The medical profession, weak and unprotected in the 19th century and the early part of the 20th century, had been steadily growing in affluence, prestige, and political power. Their lobby had become one of the most effective, if not *the* most effective, in the country. Their control of medical care was virtually unlimited. They controlled admissions to hospitals, prescription of medicines, decisions on vital issues such as operations—in short, they wielded the power of life and death, with no limits of any kind as to the amount of fees. To them, a national health program meant loss of control, lowering of income, and loss of prestige.

The AMA launched a campaign to change public opinion. The times were propitious for that. Following World War II, the Cold War had been launched by the United States, led by various committees and Senator Joseph McCarthy in a program of vilification and blacklisting of progressives in all areas. National health insurance was described as socialized medicine by the AMA. In California, Governor Earl Warren proposed a health plan of a limited kind. The AMA advertised extensively in the newspapers at the rate of $100,000 annually and was successful in defeating the Warren Plan.[6]

American Hospitals from 1946 to 1970

In August of 1946, Truman signed the Hospital Survey and Construction Act, known as the Hill-Burton Act. This was the first part of Truman's plan. It provided for grants and loans to hospitals, and nursing homes to a lesser extent, for the building and modernization of health facilities. The AMA was in favor of that.

In exchange, the recipients of the grants agreed to provide "a reasonable volume . . . of hospital service offered below cost or free, to persons unable to pay therefor . . . both legally indigent and persons who are self-supporting but are unable to pay the full cost of needed hospital care."

The passage of this Act, when added to the efforts of those opposed to national health insurance, carried the day. National health insurance, and of course socialized medicine, receded into the background. For 24 years, from the enactment of the Hill-Burton Act in 1956 to 1970, one-half of the Hill-Burton Act proceeded very actively; that is, more than 6,000 hospitals received grants totaling more than $4 billion.[7] The other half of the program, relating to the provision of free or below-cost services to those unable to pay, showed a somewhat lower level of activity. In fact, it was virtually ignored by the federal government and state agencies mandated to enforce the Act and by the recipients of these grants, namely, the hospitals and the doctors who control them.

At first there was no elucidation of the phrase "a reasonable volume" of service offered below cost or free, but eventually the Department of Health, Education, and Welfare (HEW) did set up several guidelines, 3% of cost of operations (less costs attributable to Medicare and Medicaid), or 10% per annum of the Hill-Burton grants received by the facility, whichever was less. A third option was the certification (presumably based on actuality) that the facility would turn no applicant for health service away. Still a fourth option was available. The facility could provide less service than specified in the 3% or 10% options above if it was not financially able to fulfill those options.

The New Orleans Hill-Burton Case

In 1970, the first real challenge to the way in which the free service obligation was being implemented by the state agencies and the hospitals occurred simultaneously in Colorado and Louisiana. The latter challenge is the one we are concerned with in this case study. But first we must have a little historical background, both legal and accounting in content.

Marilyn Rose, an attorney, had for several years prior to 1970 been the acting chief of the Health Branch Division of Civil Rights, Office of General Counsel of the U.S. Department of Health, Education, and Welfare (HEW) in Washington, D.C. In this capacity she learned that hospitals were violating their Hill-Burton obligations, and that no action had ever been initiated by HEW to enforce compliance. After leaving HEW prior to 1970, and joining the National Legal Program on Health Problems of the Poor, her assignment in that public interest law firm was to foster legal developments to gain access to health services for the indigent. The National Legal Program on Health Problems of the Poor later became the National Health Law Program (NHELP) and will be so designated in this study.

By this time it was apparent that HEW's interest was on a par with Ogden Nash's interest in his neighbor's children; he wrote:

> My interest in my neighbor's nursery
> Would have to improve to be even cursory.

On July 24, 1970, the New Orleans Legal Assistance Corporation together with NHELP filed a lawsuit against Ashton J. Mouton, Director of Louisiana State Department of Hospitals, and ten hospitals in New Orleans, charging them all with violating their obligations to afford adequate hospital services to persons unable to pay. During the twenty-four years since the inception of the Hill-Burton Act, the ten hospitals had received almost $15 million in Hill-Burton grants. The case was filed in the United States District Court, Eastern District of Louisiana, New Orleans Division, and is known as *Cook* v. *Ochsner Foundation Hospital* (E.D. La., Civ. No. 70–1969). The suit was later broadened to include among the defendants, Elliott Richardson, Secretary of HEW. Marilyn Rose was chief counsel for the plaintiffs.

The class action lawsuit filed on behalf of Rosezella Cook and the seven other plaintiffs maintains that all eight plaintiffs, who were seriously ill at the time of attempting to be admitted to the hospitals, were turned away for a variety of reasons, including inability to pay admission fees, test fees, examination fees by staff physicians, lack of their own physicians, valid credit cards, or hospitalization insurance. Medicaid eligibility was not considered sufficient ground for admission. Deposits were also required from indigent recipients of Medicare before admission.

The following two examples illustrate the denial process and in one case the fatal result:

Plaintiff Rosezella Cook was a 33-year-old black female, who suffers from a serious heart condition, high blood pressure, and extreme nervousness. On or about June 28, 1970, Plaintiff Cook's condition became very serious and she went to Defendant Methodist Hospital in an attempt to be admitted. She was denied admission at Defendant Methodist Hospital because she was unable to pay a deposit of $35 required of all emergency room patients by Defendants Paul B. Bjork and Methodist Hospital.

Clifford Breaux, an indigent black suffering from congestive heart failure and obesity, was denied admission to Charity Hospital on five occasions between May 5 and June 8, 1970, purportedly due to a shortage of beds. On June 10 and 11 he was refused admission to Flint Goodridge, Touro, and Ochsner hospitals since he was unable to pay the admission fee. Finally, on June 11, 1970, his brother borrowed $200 to secure his admission to Ochsner Foundation Hospital, where he died within two weeks.

The lawsuit also maintained that the defendants, in addition to denying adequate hospital services to persons unable to pay, had in all cases except one hospital, Charity Hospital (state owned), violated Title VI of the Civil Rights Act of 1964 (42 U.S.C. 2000d) and the Fourteenth Amendment of the United States Constitution by engaging in practices, policies, and customs by which persons are denied admission to facilities because of race. (All of the plaintiffs were black.) In support of its position that the hospitals with the exception of Charity Hospital had practiced discrimination, the plaintiffs' lawyers alleged that although 40% of the population of metropolitan New Orleans was black, admission data required to be submitted from these hospitals by HEW since the passage of the Civil Rights Act indicated a disproportionate number of white patients to black patients in their admissions patterns.

In 1972, two years after the lawsuit was filed, Marilyn Rose recognized that she needed accounting help. The Hill-Burton Act and the rudimentary regulations drafted to implement it, provided that facilities receiving Hill-Burton grants were obligated to furnish free or below-cost services to those unable to pay *unless it was not financially feasible for the hospital to do so.* Three of the defendant hospitals (Flint-Goodridge, Sara Mayo and Methodist) made this claim.

Rose could find no definition of *financial feasibility* in the Hill-Burton Act, the regulations implementing it, or for that matter in any other place. She tried to get help in defining it from accountants in New York City and Washington, D.C., without success. We may speculate on the reasons why this was so, but the fact is that it was. From the Urban Institute in Washington, she heard of San Francisco API (described in the preface) and applied to them for help on July 5, 1972. API quickly agreed to accept the case, after Ms. Rose had sent us financial statements and other data relating to the three hospitals.

The members of API, including the three accountants who volunteered to take primary responsibility for the case, had never seen nor heard of a definition of financial feasibility. This is not the only case in which vagueness and ambiguity characterize critical areas in federal legislation. During World War II, as an officer in the U.S. Army, I did renegotiation work for the Corps of Engineers, and in the preface I mentioned how vague had been the definition of "excessive profits. "

And so API set itself the formidable task of constructing a definition of *financial feasibility*. This case study is the story of that construction. It does more than explain the *Cook* v. *Ochsner* case; it elucidates the methodology of this type of financial analysis, and the roles played by various segments of the health delivery machinery. API had very little time to prepare its analysis, because the preliminary hearing had been set in New Orleans for July 10, 1972. What was required was an examination of the financial and other data, a determination of what financial feasibility meant in this case, and some ideas as to whether the hospitals in question were justified in claiming this defense. The mechanics of how the work was done are not the subject of this study, except to note that in addition to the three accountants assigned to the case, many other members of API contributed their ideas, and reviewed the report that was presented to API's clients, the two public interest law firms.

It is extremely important to determine what contributes to an understanding of financial feasibility. Marilyn Rose was a young, brilliant public interest lawyer, intensely interested in the medical needs of the indigent. She was the prime mover in the struggle to have the Hill-Burton Law enforced. She was also smart enough to know that she needed help in defining financial feasibility. Her chief assistant was another attorney, Jeffrey B. Schwartz, of the National Tenants Organization of Washington, D.C. There was also support from several other lawyers connected with legal assistance groups in New Orleans. On the other side of the case there was a large battalion of lawyers and administrative personnel representing the hospitals.

The task force members from API volunteering to study the accounting problems consisted of three certified public accountants: Jack Beckerman, Michael Coppersmith, and myself. Among us, we had many years of intimate knowledge of accounting concepts, auditing and accounting experience, hospital operations, and governmental health programs. In preparation for the preliminary hearing in New Orleans on July 10, 1972, the API task force, after consultation with many other members of API, wrote a report that analyzed the financial data sent to them by Marilyn Rose. The data included financial statements of the three hospitals claiming that they could not afford to provide free or below-cost service to the indigent. It also included Medicare cost reports prepared by the hospitals and other financial data and relevant legal documents. During the period immediately preceding July 10, 1972, Larry Silver, an attorney formerly with NHELP, and Jeffrey B. Schwartz, also an attorney formerly with NHELP, visited San Francisco and discussed the case with the API task force and the executive committee of API.

On July 12, in New Orleans at a conference with the three hospitals—Flint-Goodridge, Sara Mayo, and Methodist—and their attorneys, I explained our report and presented them with copies. Federal District Court Judge James A. Comiskey was also given a copy. On July 13 the hearing was held. This was not a trial, nor was there a jury, so that I was not called upon to testify. At the hearing, opening statements were made by attorneys on both sides. The judge, who seemed thoroughly conversant with API's report, more so in fact than the attorneys for the defendants, asked them a number of questions to which they responded as well as they could. On August 1, 1972, an order was issued by Judge Comiskey and consented to by all parties concerned in lieu of a trial and judgment. The defendant hospitals, seven in number at the time, agreed to provide free and below-cost service to persons unable to pay therefor in the amount of $983,000 during a fiscal year ending in 1973.

In the spring of 1974, the Cook plaintiffs claimed that six of the defendant hospitals in New Orleans had violated the settlement agreement (which had been approved by the court). Charging these defendants with contempt, attorneys for plaintiffs again sought the assistance of API. On this second occasion, I presented the API position in formal testimony and assisted plaintiffs' attorneys in analyzing the testimony of, and cross-examining, the accountant for one of the hospitals. I am treating the two hearings together, as the following discussion involves both.

The accountants for the hospitals maintained that it was not financially feasible for the hospitals to provide free care to the indigent because the hospital financial statements showed losses or small profits. Financial feasibility, however, cannot be determined solely by profit or loss statements.

It is generally assumed by the layman that an audited financial statement is correct in an absolute sense. After all, it balances and is signed by a professional who vouches for its accuracy. But let us look more closely. Certified public accountants are frequently more concerned with language than with content. When they issue a financial statement they say, "Our examination was made in accordance with *generally accepted auditing standards*." That is an interesting statement. *Generally accepted auditing standards* is a companion phrase to *generally accepted accounting principles (GAAP)*. Both of these phrases are required by the American Institute of Certified Public Accountants (AICPA). Generally accepted accounting principles! The most holy of holies! What does it mean? A great many things in recorded history have been generally accepted by large groups of people. To name a few:

"The sun revolves around the earth. People have been burned at the stake for not accepting it."
"God created the world in six days and rested on the seventh."
"The proper punishment for molesting a woman is to have your hand amputated."
"After death your soul goes to heaven, hell, or purgatory."

Consider other phrases. "*In our opinion*, the financial statements referred to above *present fairly* in all material aspects the financial position, etc."

In our opinion. Present fairly. Let us suppose that your doctor says to you, "In my opinion, it is fair to say that you have cancer." Would you accept that as a correct diagnosis?

Why is it that the phrases just discussed are so fuzzy? Because the accountant is not promising correctness. He or she is promising consistency.

Let us cite a few examples:

"Depreciation can be straight-line, accelerated in several different ways, or depreciated in still other ways. Which is correct?"
"Depreciation is usually based on the cost of the fixed asset being depreciated. The present value may be ten times cost. Is the depreciation correct?"
"Investments may be valued at cost or current value. Which is 'correct'?"
"Inventories can be valued in accordance with LIFO (last-in, first-out), FIFO (first-in, first-out), or several other methods. Are they all correct?"
"But no matter which choices the accountant makes, as long as he is consistent, the financial statements may be in accord-

ance with GAAP, however widely they vary. Right? Wrong? That is irrelevant. They are in accordance with GAAP."

Returning now to the New Orleans problem, we must recognize that an analysis of financial feasibility requires more than an acceptance of the "bottom line" profit or loss. One must examine more deeply. It should be mentioned that there were really two accounting problems presented to API. The first is the question of financial feasibility, and the second is what constitutes Hill-Burton service? I shall discuss them separately. API's definition of financial feasibility may be summarized this way:

If the hospital can afford to provide free or below-cost service to the indigent in an amount that will not endanger or hamper its operations at the time or in the future, it is financially feasible to do so, even if its financial operating statement shows a small profit or loss. This is not an abstruse or academic matter. It is a matter not of accounting complexity but of common sense. Consider the following factors:

Depreciation of Buildings

Historically, nonprofit hospitals, exempt from income tax, frequently did not record depreciation on their books because it afforded no tax advantage. With the advent of Medicare, however, this changed, because depreciation was an allowable, reimbursable cost under Title XVIII of the Social Security Act. Depreciation was allowable on a straight-line basis (1/40 of cost each year for a 40-year life, for example), or on any of several accelerated bases allowed by the Internal Revenue Service. (More than straight-line in the early years declining to less than straight-line in later years.)

Another reason for taking a close look at depreciation of buildings on the books of hospitals is that depreciation is a device to spread the cost over the life of the asset. In other words, if an organization spends $100,000 to erect a building, it would not be logical to charge all of that to the year or years during which the costs were expended. In that case, if the building is expected to last 50 years, the depreciation is 1/50 of $100,000 or $2,000 each year for 50 years. An accelerated method of depreciation would change the yearly figures, but the principle would remain the same. Suppose, however, that the organization never did incur the cost of erecting the building, but that the money was received as a grant under the Hill-Burton Act or from contributions or a combination of both. In that event, what is the rationale for considering depreciation as a yearly write-off of a cost that was never incurred by the hospital? If it is maintained that depreciation is a method of reserving funds for replacement of the building some time in the future, it is certainly relevant to ask whether the new building, too, may not be financed by government grants or private contributions. To conclude, therefore, depreciation of a building does not require the present outlay of funds and may never require such an outlay. In that event, one may question whether its inclusion as an operating expense on the financial statements of the hospital may be relevant from the point of view of financial feasibility.

It should also be noted that when the hospitals were reimbursed by the federal government for costs incurred in the treatment of Medicare patients, depreciation was included in costs. And now, to cap it all, the depreciation expense is again used to claim that it reduces profit, and therefore precludes free or below-cost services to the indigent. A triple play may be a rarity in baseball (only one has ever happened in World Series games, and that was decades ago), but hospitals perform it frequently.

Fixed and Variable Expenses

Certain expenses, such as administrative salaries, various other salaries, professional fees, insurance and interest, are fixed or relatively fixed. That is, relatively small increases in service will not increase such expenses or will increase them very slightly. Other expenses, such as postage, food, supplies, linen, etc., are variables; that is, they will increase in proportion to increases in service rendered. Let us consider a hypothetical case:

Fixed Expenses	$1,500,000
Variable Expenses	500,000
Total Expenses	$2,000,000
Beds	150
In-patient Days	35,000
Occupancy	64%

In this case the hospital can easily accommodate more patients, since the occupancy rate of 64% is below optimal capacity (usually considered to be 85%). The cost of providing one day of in-patient care on an overall basis is slightly over $57.00 ($2,000,000 divided by the number of in-patient days, 35,000). Since most of the expenses are fixed, however, it should be noted that care could be provided to additional in-patients at an additional cost of slightly over $14.00 per day ($500,000 divided by the number of in-patient days, 35,000).

The significance of this calculation is that the hospital is offered several methods of providing free or below-cost service without being subjected to financial hardship. Since there are vacant beds, service could be provided to indigent patients for about $14.00 per day, or half of the indigent patients could be provided service for $28.00 per day and the other half free. Obviously, there are many combinations that could be effected to provide free or below-cost service to indigent patients with no net cost or relatively little net cost to the hospital.

This concept was formulated by Clark C. Havighurst, professor of law at Duke University, in an article that reflects work supported by Health Services Research Center, Inter-Study, Minneapolis. He stated: "It is widely accepted that an empty stand-by bed costs about two-thirds as much as an occupied one. This implies that a bed, once it is in being, should be used if the value of hospitalization to the patient is at least one-third the total cost to the hospital."[8]

Noncash Expenses

It may be quite correct from an accounting point of view to claim that certain expenses can reduce net income on a financial statement but still should be excluded from the standpoint of financial feasibility. Consider two such items that were relevant in the present case. One was the abandonment of an old building after a new hospital had been built. The book value of the abandoned building, let us say $100,000, was written off and reduced income by that amount. Did that limit the ability of the hospital to provide free service? Not at all. No maintenance money was spent on the abandoned building during the year of abandonment. That $100,000 should be added to net income when considering financial feasibility. The same thing is true in the case of loss on the sale of old equipment.

Following are several examples of incorrect statements by the hospitals concerning Hill-Burton service:

Hill-Burton Law and regulations require prior determination

(except in the case of emergency) for service to be considered valid. In other words, at the time of admission to the hospital, it shall be decided by the hospital that the patient be given free or below-cost service. However, some of the hospitals claimed bad debts, in one case going back six years, as valid Hill-Burton compliance. This is clearly illegal. It is equivalent to stating that a department store's bad debts constitute charitable contributions, which of course is absurd.

One of the more bizarre claims was made by the Hotel Dieu Hospital. They claimed that a new out-patient clinic had been built specifically to serve Hill-Burton patients. They claimed that the cost of running it for the year amounted to $38,390 and that fees were received in the amount of $2,057. The excess of cost ($38,390 less $2,057) was $36,333 and that, they claimed, was Hill-Burton compliance.

If we accept that interpretation we would logically have to accept the following:

	Per Hospital	10% More Service	10% Less Service	No Service
Total Clinic Cost	$38,390	$38,390	$38,390	$38,390
Revenue to Clinic	2,057	2,263	1,851	0
Hill-Burton Service	$36,333	$36,127	$36,539	$38,390

In other words, the more patients seen and the more revenue collected, the less Hill-Burton service claimed, and vice versa. When I demonstrated this on the blackboard in court, even the judge and the defendants' attorneys were amused.

As mentioned earlier, the first hearing was held on July 13, 1972. On August 1, 1972, a consent court order was signed by Judge Comiskey, attorneys for the plaintiffs, and representatives of the defendant hospitals. It ordered the defendant hospitals to provide free and below-cost services to persons unable to pay therefor, in differing amounts for each hospital, the total being $983,000. Another very important provision of the order was the requirement that in connection with the provision of free and below-cost services, said hospitals shall make prior determinations of eligibility for services. This, however, was followed by the ubiquitous phrase "when feasible."

The medical professionals acted as though they had never heard of the Hill-Burton Law even though they had been the greatest beneficiaries of it for 25 years. The exclusion of potential Hill-Burton clients was clearly their responsibility because only physicians can admit patients to the hospitals. Refusal to admit potential Hill-Burton patients when the obligation is clearly present constitutes a simple case of law-breaking.

There is no doubt that the Hill-Burton Act did modernize many health care facilities and built many new ones, resulting in improved, though more expensive medical care for those able to afford it. But to what extent did it benefit the indigent? As we have seen, they were systematically refused admittance to hospitals, even though they were grievously ill. *The billions of dollars expended by the federal government went not for health care for the indigent, for whose benefit the Hill-Burton Law was enacted, but to the health care providers.*

In a city whose metropolitan population is over one million, free or below-cost service of $983,000 is obviously a drop in the bucket. Nevertheless, the consequences were momentous:

1. For the first time since the inception of the Hill-Burton Law, now in its 26th year, it was being enforced.
2. For the first time, there was an attempt to define financial feasibility. This would give some guidance to lawyers attempting to bring about enforcement of the law. It would also enable HEW and the state bodies responsible for the enforcement of the law to administer it intelligently.
3. The successful cooperation of legal and accounting disciplines emphasized the need for and the effectiveness of an interdisciplinary approach to the solution of public interest matters.

In conclusion, I wish to call attention to the role of the actors in this drama.

The accounting profession, prior to the Cook case, ignored the Hill-Burton Act, even though the audits performed by CPA firms normally require an examination of legal obligations of the audited entity (hospital) and a verification of compliance with obligations. Many audited reports now comment on Hill-Burton compliance, although it is notable that the ATCPA's *Hospital Audit Guide,* Fourth Edition, 1982, makes no mention of Hill-Burton in the text, sample financial statements or notes to financial statements. The accounting firms satisfied their professional responsibilities by preparing audited statements in accordance with GAAP, but managed to obscure the financial feasibility issue both in their statements and in their testimony at the hearings. One of the CPAs testifying for one of the hospitals stated that there was no clear distinction between fixed and variable expenses, citing the example of interest rates that may change from year to year. This statement would be apparent nonsense to anyone who has the most elementary knowledge of accounting or budgeting. The lawyers representing the hospitals defended all of the hospitals' misrepresentations. After all, who pays their fees? The hospitals prior to the case never considered Hill-Burton compliance a legal or moral requirement even though they had eagerly accepted the grants. They claimed bad debts as Hill-Burton compliance in complete disregard of the law and even claimed that the entire cost of a clinic constituted Hill-Burton compliance although it rendered practically no service to indigents. They also sought the shelter of lack of financial feasibility where it was nonexistent. The federal and state governments, mandated to enforce the law, were completely moribund and derelict in their duties.

Hill-Burton—Nashville, Tennessee

In the case of *Cook* v. *Ochsner*, discussed previously, the issue was one of financial feasibility—could the hospitals afford to provide free or below-cost service in the required amount? In the case I am about to discuss, we confront a different problem—prior determination. What that means will become clear as we proceed with the case of Callie Mae Newsom, on her own behalf and on the behalf of all others similarly situated, Plaintiff v. Professional Adjustment Services, Inc.; Vanderbilt University; Mary Jane Livingston and Eugene W. Fowinkle, M.D. (both of Vanderbilt University Hospital); Caspar Weinberger, Secretary of HEW; Defendants. This was heard before Honorable L. Clure Morton, United States District Judge of the Middle District of Tennessee, Nashville District.

I first learned of the case from Andreas Schneider of the National Health Law Program (NHELP) in a letter addressed to API, October 11, 1976. He stated that he had been asked to assist Gordon Bonnyman of Nashville Legal Services to try the case of *Newsom* v. *Professional Adjustment Service*. The case was a federal class action suit for injunctive and declaratory relief against Vanderbilt Medical Center, its collection agency, the Tennessee Hill-Burton Agency and DHEW.

The central issue of the suit was whether Vanderbilt Medical Center had violated its "uncompensated services" assurance by billing and suing persons unable to pay, without giving them an opportunity to apply for free or below-cost services. Schneider requested API to assist in analyzing the discovery materials on this point in preparation for trial.

Accountants for the Public Interest, for reasons not relevant here, was unable to accept the case, but it was accepted by me personally in my capacity as a certified public accountant.

Within a few days I had reason to regret my decision. I was buried under an avalanche of paper. Lawyers Bonnyman and Schneider operated on the theory that the scales of justice were tipped in the direction of the side with the greater documentary avoirdupois. There were financial statements, both audited and un-audited, published brochures, depositions, Medicare cost reports, interoffice correspondence, various legal memoranda, organization charts, copies of communications between counsel on both sides, copies of the Hill-Burton Act and regulations, notes by the attorneys on all of the above, duplicate copies of some of the above and occasionally triplicates. Because some of these documents covered several years, it was a formidable task simply to look at it all; forming an accounting opinion of it was even more formidable.

There was no dispute as to the amount of federal grants received by the hospital pursuant to the Hill-Burton Act for construction projects initiated between 1957 and 1971: $3,181,009.63. The hospital elected to provide, on an annual basis, a volume of "uncompensated services" to "persons unable to pay" equal to 10% of the grants received, or $318,101. I met with Schneider and subsequently with him and Bonnyman. Both of them were extremely intelligent, capable, and expert in legal aspects of Hill-Burton, but they felt a little out of their depth when confronted with accounting problems. They had already taken depositions from several of the key people at Vanderbilt Hospital, and as I have mentioned, had amassed materials, copies of which they gave to me. I promptly waded through them.

On November 16, 1976, I wrote to Mr. Bonnyman, concluding the letter as follows:

It appears that Vanderbilt University Hospital has not complied with HEW regulations re Hill-Burton uncompensated care because:
1. The hospital made no prior determinations.
2. They furnished possible Hill-Burton clients with no notices equivalent to the required posted notices.
3. Alleged Hill-Burton service appears to be bad-debt write-offs and not Hill-Burton service.

It appears that neither HEW nor the Tennessee Department of Public Health monitored or enforced Hill-Burton regulations in this case because:

1. They did not investigate 1, 2, and 3 above.
2. They had no adequate figures to determine alleged Hill-Burton compliance.

This letter did not come out of the blue. It followed my study of depositions of Mr. Hewitt Rogers, Director of Admissions, and Mr. George C. Forsyth, Director of Financial Management of Vanderbilt Hospital. The Hill-Burton Regulations state, "There shall be included only those services (Hill-Burton) provided to an individual with respect to whom the applicant has made a written determination prior to the provision of such services that such an individual is unable to pay therefor . . . " Both of the depositions make it very clear that no such prior determinations were made or even considered. On the contrary, when asked whether the patient was ever told he could be considered for uncompensated care, Mr. Rogers replied: "Well, if you're interviewing me for admission and if I have the possibility of payment and you tell me that I would be considered for uncompensated responsibilities, you would diminish my willingness to pay very greatly." To put it bluntly, the answer is no, we do not advise them of the possibility of obtaining uncompensated care.

Mr. Forsyth carried it one step further. He said he was not aware that the Vanderbilt Medical Center had received any Hill-Burton money. As he said, it "really wasn't an issue until I heard of the involvement of the organization you represent in a suit." *A federal law enacted 30 years prior to this statement was not an issue to the director of financial management of the hospital.*

Mr. Forsyth's deposition is also interesting because of the discussion of what we may call the Bucket Theory of Accounting, page 29. This is not only a lucid description of a non existent accounting theory, but also displays a fine administrative sensibility to patients. At one point he says:

Therefore there are a great many patients who receive free service and whom we know will be free service and particularly, anyone in that category who comes into the emergency room we try to avoid having them bleeding all over the floor while we get the financial information and also outpatients where there is no financial screening process, anyone in that category will merely get thrown into the bad debt bucket, which is not a literal definition or description.

Needless to say, Mr. Forsyth is not suggesting that the patient should get thrown into the bucket. He is implying that the charge for that person's medical care will be entered into the Hill-Burton account on the books of the hospital. It is also noteworthy that his statement might have been written by a retarded fourth-grade child.

The Trial

Although the trial was originally scheduled to take place late in 1976, it was delayed several times because of the judge's busy schedule. On one occasion I was enroute to Nashville to testify as an expert witness, when I was paged at the San Francisco Airport and told of the delay. Eventually, on September 8, 1977, the trial was held. Representing the plaintiff were Gordon Bonnyman of the Legal Services of Nashville, Inc., and Andreas Schneider of National Health Law Program (NHELP). Representing the hospital was Attorney William Ozier. Attorney William Farmer was there on behalf of HEW, assisted by Attorney Carol Conrad, and Attorney C. Hayes Cooney represented the State of Tennessee. I was present as an expert witness.

At the trial, one witness, Mr. Edward Lee Green, 68 years of age, testified that he had an ulcerated stomach and that one night he started to vomit blood. Because he was a resident of Cheatham County, which had no hospital, his son took him to the emergency room at Vanderbilt Hospital. He said that the doctor run (sic) a tube down his nose into his stomach and then asked what kind of insurance he had. On hearing that the patient had no health insurance and was on Social Security, the doctor replied, "Well, you can't go to General Hospital because you live in Cheatham County, and we can't keep you because you've got no insurance. Saint Thomas takes cases like you."

Green testified further that he was too sick to see any signs relating to the hospital's obligation to provide charity care to indigent patients and nobody told him about that.

Another witness, Mrs. Blanche Mary Darnell, 37 years of age, of Chapel Hill, Tennessee, was sent to Vanderbilt Hospital by Dr. Everett Howell. The reason for the referral was that she had been in a car wreck and was having back trouble, neck trouble, headaches, pains in her arm, loss of feeling in some of her fingers, and it was her doctor's opinion that she needed tests and X-rays. She then explained that the estimated length of stay in the hospital was 10 days, and that if she didn't have insurance to cover the stay she would have to pay 900 dollars on admittance and the balance (amount undisclosed) when dismissed. She noticed no signs about the Hill-Burton obligation, was not told of it, was not advised of availability at any other hospital, and was not admitted because she could not pay.

Several other patients testified and then I was put on the stand. Basically my testimony set forth some of the legal basis for the suit:[9]

Uncompensated services consist of four types. [Before describing them, let me explain that hospital accounting requires that *all* services be billed originally at full service price on the books. Uncompensated services are treated as deductions.]

1. Courtesy allowances arising from discounts offered to employees of the hospital, or to their relatives.
2. Contract allowances representing the difference between, for example, Medicare billings and Medicare payments received. If billings exceed payments received, the difference is considered uncompensated service.
3. Bad debts constitute a third type. If uncollected they are written off as an expense.
4. When a hospital receives Hill-Burton funds, it agrees to provide a reasonable volume of free or below-cost care to the indigent. The amount below normal charges is uncompensated care. *That is what we are concerned with in this case.*

Under the Hill-Burton program, the uncompensated care must be determined prior to admittance of the patient to the hospital.[10] This is not a new concept, because the American Institute of CPAs has put out a manual called *The Hospital Audit Guide,*[11] which spells out the same sort of principle, and the *Chart of Accounts* put out by the American Hospital Association, which is a definitive study from an accounting point of view, also makes the same point. These two spell out that prior determination must be made. That is to say, when the patient comes in, it must be determined whether or not that patient can pay. If the hospital is a Hill-Burton institution and has received Hill-Burton grants or loans, the hospital has to furnish a certain dollar amount of such care and must make prior determination. There are, however, two exceptions to this.[12] One is in the case of emergency care where prior determination cannot be made until later because it would be at the expense, possibly, of the patient's life. The other is the case when the patient, when admitted, was expected to incur a cost of, let us say, $1000, and the actual cost turned out to be $10,000. The patient could have paid $1000 but could not pay the $10,000. In that event, that is the second exception. It may be determined then that this is an uncompensated Hill-Burton obligation—the unpaid portion. However, it should be noted that these are exceptions and not the rule, and they are spelled out as such in the regulations issued by HEW.

Then I was asked to comment on the admission policy of the hospital. Mr. Schneider presented me with a document and the testimony proceeded as follows:

Q: Could you describe this document, please, sir?

A: This is Vanderbilt University Hospital's weekly summary of patients denied admission for financial reasons, week ending 8:00 a.m., Monday, October the 11th.

It includes 21 items describing or giving the name of the patient, the physician requesting admission, the clinical services needed, the date admission was denied, and it says in the last column, "Patient referred for care to," and then it has a description of why the patient was denied service and what referral was made for some other source.

Q: Mr. Coleman, was this one of the documents that you reviewed in rendering your opinion that Vanderbilt University Hospital was not in compliance with the Hill-Burton program?

A: Yes.

Q: And what in this document led you to that conclusion?

A: Well, this is what I called prior determination of a different kind, and that is determination that because the patient did not have enough insurance or enough money he would not be admitted.

For example, some of the entries go like this, "No insurance. Could not make deposit. Refer to Nashville General."

"Insufficient insurance. Refer to Nashville General."

"Used all but five days Medicare and has old balance of $41,000. Refer to Vocational Rehabilitation."

"Insufficient insurance. To come at a later date."

"No insurance. Clear," et cetera.

This is prior determination, but it's a determination not to render charity service.

I was then asked to determine whether financial statements issued by Vanderbilt University Hospital could substantiate the amount of Hill-Burton uncompensated services that had been provided to persons unable to pay therefor. I had examined those statements and answered that the statements comingled charity allowance (Hill-Burton) with other uncompensated services described above, so that there was no way to ascertain the amount of Hill-Burton uncompensated service.

The Decision

On June 1, 1978, approximately nine months after the trial, Judge Morton issued a large erudite memorandum on the case and a contemporaneous order to Vanderbilt Hospital, based on the memorandum. The following quotation from the memorandum states the judge's opinion of HEW's performance and the hospital's compliance. Footnote references have been eliminated.

> HEW's shortcomings in enforcing compliance with the free care provision of the Hill-Burton Act, attributed by one authority to "the tendency of regulatory agencies to become the 'captive' of the viewpoint of the very interests they were intended to regulate," has created problems in determining just what constitutes compliance. The free service obligation was virtually ignored until 1972, 25 years after Hill-Burton was enacted and 15 years after Vanderbilt received its first grant. . . .
>
> The evidence before the court in this case (some of which contradicts the factual bases assigned by the Secretary for his finding of Vanderbilt's compliance) establishes that if the current interpretation of the meaning of "compliance" were applied retroactively, Vanderbilt would be found seriously wanting. The court agrees that at least until very recently Vanderbilt at best regarded its Hill-Burton obligation as a final write-off for bad debts and at worst ignored it completely.

Eventually Judge Morton issued an order stating that Vanderbilt University Hospital was to submit reports of the reasonable cost of services rendered by it for each fiscal year from July 1, 1973, to the then-current date. The reports were to include only true Hill-Burton uncompensated services duly qualified by affidavit. Other technical matters were mentioned, but the gist of the order was clear.

As everyone expected, Vanderbilt Hospital appealed the decision to the Sixth Circuit Court of Appeals. I do not intend to quote extensively from the Court of Appeals decision, but I cannot refrain from discussing two points. One of the comments in the decision reads as follows:

> This Court has made an independent review of the legislative history of the Hill-Burton Act and must conclude that the history of the 1946 Act, in which the reasonable volume assurances first appeared, does not indicate that Congress necessarily wanted the hospitals to provide free services and thereby take care of the indigent and it surely did not intend to create a right to free services to those indigents residing in the territorial area serviced by the hospital.

This may be crystal clear to the judicial mind, but, not being a judge, I had difficulty with it. Finally I realized I had the wrong perspective. If the reader will kindly bear with me, we shall step through the looking glass and join Alice In Wonderland, who has just begun a conversation with the White Queen.

"Off with their heads!" shouted the White Queen.

"You can't do that," said Alice in horror, "The law says decapitation is illegal."

"Nonsense," said the Queen. "The law doesn't say anything. Do you know what a spoon is, Child?"

"Of course," answered Alice. "What has that to do with it?"

"Does a spoon say anything?" asked the Queen.

"Of course not!" replied Alice. "A spoon is a thing. It can't say anything."

"And what is a law?" said the Queen triumphantly. "It's a thing."

"Then how can you tell what a law means?" inquired Alice.

"It's a thing. It doesn't mean anything. We have to find out what the lawmakers intended."

"And how do you do that?" asked Alice.

"Off with their heads!" shouted the Queen.

"Why?" shouted Alice in return.

"Because," said the Queen, "if we cut off their heads we can look inside and see what their intentions were. You didn't think you would find their intentions in their feet, did you?"

"But suppose some of the lawmakers are dead?" asked Alice, who was beginning to get confused.

"O that!" said the Queen. "That's a posthumous matter."

Alice thought a posthume was something like a costume, but she wasn't sure.

"But if 75 lawmakers voted for the law and 25 against it, how can you tell what *the* intention of the lawmakers was?" asked Alice.

The Queen turned to the Judge. "Off with her head!" she screamed. "She asks too many questions."

With that quotation clarified, we can proceed to another:

19. Constitutional Law 252.5. No member of class fitting qualifications of indigency for purposes of Hill-Burton free care in hospital, merely by being member of class, had any right to such free services and which class members would be benefitted was left solely to discretion of hospital as long as minimum amount was provided; thus, although the class might have the right to have hospital give benefits to some of class members and thus have standing under the statute, no individual had legitimate claim to free services such that procedures provided would infringe a due process right. U.S.C.A. Const. Amends. 5, 14; Public Health Service Act, s 603(e) as amended 42 U.S.C.A. s 291c(e); Hospital Survey and Construction Act, s 601, 60 Stat. 1040.

Once more we step through the looking glass to join Alice in Wonderland and the White Queen.

"Let's play a game," said the Queen to Alice.

"I love games," replied Alice. "What's the name of the game?"

"Going to the hospital," answered the Queen. "I am the doctor who admits people to the hospital, or refuses to admit them."

As Alice looked, the Queen slowly changed into a male doctor in a white coat. A stethoscope hung around his neck.

"You are an indigent, black, sick, dying patient," said the doctor. "You want to be admitted to the hospital for treatment. Start the game."

"I want to get into the hospital," said Alice.

"And who are you?"

"I am an indigent."

"So?"

"I am sick," said Alice.

"That's what they all say."

"I am so sick I am dying," responded Alice. "And it says here that you should admit some sick indigents."

"Yes," said the doctor slyly, "but no *one* indigent has the right to get in."

"But have you already admitted all the indigents you were supposed to admit for this year?" asked Alice.

"No," said the doctor, "but if you have a legitimate claim to free services you would infringe my due process right. Do you have any money, like $7,325.14?"

"No."

"Then," said the doctor, "please go away. Besides, you are bleeding all over the floor. Here's a bucket and a mop. Clean the floor on the way out."

Alice looked at the doctor more closely. It was changing. The white coat and stethoscope disappeared. Very slowly it developed four stubby legs, a snout and a thin, curly tail. It looked at Alice with tiny, mischievous eyes and trotted away.

On June 25, 1981, Judge Morton issued an Agreed Order, by which Vanderbilt Hospital was to deliver $1,141,041.50 of free service for the fiscal years 1973–74, as "remedial obligation" that they had failed to deliver for those two years. The following three years, as the amount was undetermined, were to be adjusted after the necessary data was accumulated by the hospital.

On October 10, 1982, Gordon Bonnyman and Russell G. Averby of Legal Services of Middle Tennessee, Inc., filed a *Brief in Support of Plaintiffs' Motion to Hold the Defendant Vanderbilt University in Contempt of Court*. At the same time the legal firm also filed *Plaintiffs' Brief in Support of the Motion to Adjudicate Vanderbilt University's Hill-Burton Deficit for Fiscal Year 1976–1978*. The latter brief included a computation that the hospital's obligation for the three years amounted to $1,700,000. According to the same brief, Vanderbilt Hospital, after numerous changes, claims to have fulfilled $227,000 of its Hill-Burton obligation for the same three years. Both briefs emphasize the constant changes in hospital claims of Hill-Burton services and various abuses in denying service to indigents, illegal billing and collection efforts, denial of due process, failure to notify patients of their rights, and in general a complete disregard of the law.

The final action on the case came on March 23, 1983, when

Judge Morton, after eight years, issued *Newsom*'s last order and opinion. In them he reversed his previous opinion and refused to hold Vanderbilt Hospital in contempt. He denied attorney's fees to the plaintiffs. He determined the amount of Hill-Burton uncompensated care that the hospital failed to provide as $2,240,633 for the five years ended in 1978, and ordered the hospital to make up that much as remedial care. He then considered the case "retired."

Once more the actors in the drama play their roles. The federal and state agencies, as mentioned by the judge, have displayed a total lack of interest in enforcing an Act that is intended to provide health care for the indigent. Vanderbilt Hospital hotly defends its lack of compliance with the law and is aided and abetted by lawyers. Certified public accountants in their audit statements did nothing to ascertain compliance. The court of appeals explains how the hospital can refuse to comply with the law. The judge finally agrees with the court of appeals. The doctors are busy refusing to admit dying indigent people.

In the preceding chapter, we noted that in New Orleans the hospitals evaded their Hill-Burton obligations by refusing to render uncompensated service, because, as they erroneously claimed, it was not financially feasible to do so.

Here, in Nashville, Vanderbilt also evaded its Hill-Burton obligation, erroneously claiming that bad debts were not business losses but charity service, in spite of regulations to the contrary.

As Alphonse Karr said in 1849, "Plus ça change, plus c'est la même chose." (The more things change, the more they remain the same.)

Lastly, it should be observed that in spite of the two cases, the Hill-Burton Law is still very inadequately enforced.

2. County Hospitals—an Endangered Species

In Chapter 1, I discussed the history of American hospitals, concentrating primarily on the Hill-Burton Act of 1946, and the failure of the hospitals to provide free or below-cost service to the indigent in flagrant disregard of their legal obligation. Those hospitals were private, whether nonprofit or proprietary. Now, however, I shall discuss some of the problems of the government-run county hospitals. They were not involved in the Hill-Burton problem, because they did not have a choice when it came to serving the indigent. For example, California in its Welfare and Institutions Code, Section 17000, states that:

> Every county and every city and county shall relieve and support all incompetent, poor, indigent persons, and those incapacitated by age, disease, or accident, lawfully resident herein, when such persons are not supported and relieved by their relatives or friends, by their own means or by state hospitals or either state or private institutions.

Most of the county hospitals in the other states had similar requirements. Although private hospitals did frequently provide care to the indigent in cases of emergency, their general approach was to admit a few poor people but refer most of them to county hospitals, a practice that came to be known by the unsavory term "patient dumping." In essence we had a simple scenario: the indigent to the county hospitals, the well-to-do to private hospitals. Until the advent of Medicare and Medicaid (Medi-Cal in California) in 1965, this arrangement was satisfactory to private hospitals, whether nonprofit or proprietary.

Advent of Medicare and Medicaid

In 1965, however, we saw the beginning of a new ball game. Millions of people who formerly were unable to pay or who had no health insurance became eligible for Medicare and Medicaid, and the federal or state governments, respectively, paid for services covered by those programs. The private nonprofit and proprietary hospitals made every effort to admit patients who could pay or who were covered by third-party payment sources, whether government or private. Nonpaying or noncovered patients were shunted off to county hospitals.

A number of other complicating forces were at work at the same time. Hospitals were becoming underoccupied, as the result of shorter hospital stays by patients, overbuilding of hospital facilities in part as a consequence of Hill-Burton grants, and in some cases because of denial of service to those who needed hospital care but could not arrange for payment.

County hospitals, operating at a loss in practically all cases because they were obligated to treat patients who could not pay, were sources of embarrassment to county officials, who were criticized for allowing the unavoidable losses to occur.

Several strategies were developed to deal with this problem. One was to contract with hospital management firms to run county hospitals, in the hope that they could introduce efficiencies and operate in the absence of political pressure. Another approach was to have the county hospital contract with other providers to handle specific services, such as pediatrics, obstetrics, etc. A third method of attack was to close the county hospital and depend on private hospitals to take care of the indigent.

As perceived by neighborhood groups and organizations interested in helping the indigent get adequate care, all three of these approaches had serious weaknesses. There were fears that the poor would be dunned for bills they could not pay, and hence would be discouraged from seeking hospital admissions. There were concerns that private hospitals would be so involved in running a fiscally solvent operation that they would bypass the poor. Some people felt, and not without reason, that the private hospitals had been conditioned through the years to favor the paying patient more than the indigent.

Until the early 1970s, county hospitals covered most of California. By 1975, eight county hospitals open in 1971 had been closed, five county hospitals previously operated by the counties had their status changed and were managed by private corporations, and closure was a threat to many more.[1] The Yolo County Hospital was one of the latter group.

Hospital Closure Attempt—Yolo County, California

Yolo County is situated near Sacramento, the capital of California. It is an agricultural community with three hospitals: Woodland Memorial, a private nonprofit hospital with a bed capacity of 210; Davis Community Hospital, with a bed capacity of 48; and Yolo County Hospital, with a bed capacity of 114. In February, 1976, an ad hoc committee appointed by the Yolo County Board of Supervisors issued a detailed document entitled *Report on Consolidation of Hospital Services*. It called for a public hearing in May, 1976. The general tenor of the report was that from every point of view, closing the county hospital was desirable. Among other things, better medical care would be provided, a number of empty beds would be eliminated, and efficiencies could be introduced.

The people in the community, however, did not see it that way. The first hearing held on Tuesday evening, May 4, 1976, was described by the newspaper *The Daily Democrat* as follows:

> More than 450 filled the Home Arts Building at the Yolo County Fairgrounds Tuesday evening to voice strident objection to closing Yolo General Hospital. . . .
> Before adjourning at 11 p.m., 32 people had spoken and all but three were direct and enthusiastic in their support of Yolo General.

The Commission on Aging, former patients of Yolo General Hospital, Dr. Thomas Bodenheimer, coauthor of "Closing the Doors on the Poor" (a report on public hospital closures throughout California), the Sacramento Legal Aid Society, an intern at Yolo General Hospital, the Economic Opportunity Commission Board, and many others opposed the closure.

In 1976, the Legal Aid Society of Sacramento County, California, requested Accountants for the Public Interest (API) to perform some fiscal analysis in connection with the proposed closure of Yolo General Hospital. The Society felt that such a closure would adversely affect the poor population of the county for several reasons. In the first place, in California, county hospitals are legally bound to provide medical care to the poor, whereas private hospitals are not. In the second place, there was reason to believe that if Yolo General Hospital should be closed, Woodland Memorial Hospital, which was being proposed as the substitute health provider, might not provide free or below-cost care to the indigent.[2] In addition, the Legal Aid Society explained that it could not understand the documents suggesting the necessity for closure of Yolo General.

API was asked by the Legal Aid Society to respond to the following three questions:

1. Is the operating deficit claimed for Yolo General supportable by the data contained in the financial statements and related documents?[3]
2. Has there been any misinterpretation of accounting data by the ad hoc committee in reaching its conclusion to recommend the closing of Yolo General Hospital?
3. Has Woodland Memorial met its obligation to render a reasonable amount of free and part-pay care under the Hill-Burton Act?

The answer to both 1 and 2 was that basically the numbers used were not documented sufficiently; that the comparison of actual data for past periods and projected data for future periods were inadequately explained, and in some cases undated; that marginal corrections in the reports were not supported; and that, in general, the conclusions were extremely confusing.

As to the third question about Hill-Burton compliance, it is necessary to refer to the regulations promulgated by HEW. There are three methods of compliance stipulated.[4]

* Free or below-cost service to the indigent equal to 10% of Hill-Burton grants;
* Free or below-cost service to the indigent equal to 3% of the hospital's operating cost; or
* The hospital will not deny admission to anyone unable to pay.

The answer to the 10% option is as follows:

Estimated Hill-Burton grants to Woodland Memorial[5]	$969,000
10% thereof (rounded to thousands)	$97,000

The answer to the 3% option is as follows:

Net cost of operations, year ended 9/30/75[6] $5,186,787
Less: Medicare and Medi-Cal reimbursements[7] $2,385,922
 Net cost of operations $2,800,865
3% thereof (rounded to thousands) $84,000

In summary then we have:

10% compliance amount $97,000
3% compliance amount $84,000
Charity allowance (Hill-Burton) per Woodland Memorial $6,000

It is obvious that the 10% and the 3% options were not met.

The option chosen by Woodland Memorial Hospital was not to deny admission to anyone unable to pay (open door policy).[8] Woodland Memorial made this choice on January 30, 1976, by so certifying to the California Health Facilities Commission. *However, the Legal Aid Society had written affidavits and newspaper accounts of individuals stating that they had been denied admission to Woodland Memorial.*

An issue closely related to the matter of Hill-Burton compliance by Woodland Memorial Hospital is the apparent lack of a mechanism in the ad hoc committee report to assure the admission and treatment of the indigent population. This mechanism or procedure is necessary for Woodland Memorial with the closing of Yolo General. The following statements are taken from pages 28 and 29 of the ad hoc committee report (emphasis supplied):

- Those specialty physicians *wishing* to attend and/or treat Medi-Cal and County indigent patients admitted from the County clinic *should be willing* to work in the County outpatient clinic *if requested,* in the interest of continuity of care.
- Patients of the County outpatient clinic who need hospitalization *can be admitted* to a participating hospital on an elective basis by the County clinic physician *assuming* he has obtained medical staff privileges. He *might* also refer the patient to another physician or hospital *at his option.*

These quotations constitute fine examples of misleading political bombast. *Wishing, should be willing, if requested, can be admitted, assuming, might, at his option.* All of these things refer to what the physician might do if, if, and if. If not, forget it! One looks in vain for mention of the patients' rights.

After the first public hearing, the Board of Supervisors voted unanimously to keep Yolo General Hospital open. Although this appears to be a clear-cut victory for the community, it may not be permanent. The danger always exists that the closure issue may be revived. To underscore the problem, it should be noted that between 1964 and 1980, 28 California county hospitals were terminated. Twenty-nine counties in California had no county hospitals in 1980.

The whole Yolo episode once again illustrates the attempt of the organized medical profession and the hospitals, in this case with the initial support of the Board of Supervisors of the county, to erode the health delivery system for the indigent. The lawyer for the hospital initially maintained that the hospital (Woodland) had complied with Hill-Burton. Later he changed his position. Once more the accounting profession ignored the Hill-Burton Act.

The severity of the problem is accelerating.[9] On January 29, 1991, the National Association of Public Hospitals reported that city hospitals (county) have deteriorated during the past decade and desperately need an adequate supply of money to take care of the poor, the uninsured, the indigent, drug abuse, and AIDS patients.[10] The absence of additional funds will increase the numbers of such people, prevent prenatal care, increase disease and crime, and result in greater health care costs, welfare costs, and law enforcement costs—to say nothing of human suffering.

Sometimes, county hospital closure was attempted openly, as in Yolo County, but sometimes the issue was approached more subtly, as in Fresno County, California, which we are about to examine.

Hospital Management Firms—
Fresno County, California

The Valley Medical Center of Fresno (VMC) is a county hospital in the state of California. It is situated in the city of Fresno and is governed by such bylaws as a majority vote of the Fresno County Board of Supervisors adopts and approves. It provides preventive, diagnostic, curative, and restorative health care to inpatients and outpatients. It is also a teaching hospital; that is to say, it has a comprehensive educational program that prepares doctors who may subsequently practice not only in the community, but far beyond the confines of the county and state. Like all hospitals that are subdivisions of political entities, it always loses money because it serves all who apply whether they can afford to pay or not. Consequently, like similar hospitals elsewhere, it is under constant political pressure to economize, improve its efficiency, and at least break even if it cannot show a profit. For this reason it is an obvious target for hospital management firms, who promise to improve the fiscal operation of the hospital for a fee. Although there may be variations in each case, these firms supply management and advisory personnel on a full- or part-time basis, data processing services and purchasing services on a shared basis, etc.

On November 16, 1979, the Community Coalition on Valley Medical Center (of Fresno) wrote to Accountants for the Public Interest (API) soliciting its help in analyzing the fiscal soundness of recommendations from several quarters in Fresno County, California, that the county hospital, Valley Medical Center, should be operated under contract with one of the various companies that have entered the lucrative field of hospital management in recent years. The 1975–1976 Fresno County Grand Jury had recommended to the Superior Court and to the Board of Supervisors, which in turn requested the Chief Administrative Officer (CAO) to undertake a study to ascertain the financial feasibility of such a step. The CAO then sent requests for preliminary proposals to fifteen private firms that had indicated an initial interest.

Eventually the field boiled down to two firms, National Medical Enterprises, Inc. (NME) and Hyatt Medical Management Services, Inc. (Hyatt). The requested proposals were to be submitted in late February or March, 1980, after they had visited the hospital. The CAO at that time was to present their evaluations of the proposals based on a review by a committee composed of two CAO staff and two county hospital administrators located elsewhere in California.

The Community Coalition on Valley Medical Center was composed of a group of organizations and individuals that came together to study public versus private management of the county hospital and their actual and potential impact on availability and quality of services to the VMC patients. The coalition had explored many of the same sources of information investigated by the grand jury, as well as some additional sources, and had tentatively concluded that there was substantial reason to doubt that private management would be beneficial to the San Joaquin community that uses the services of VMC, especially the low-income people who were frequently unable to obtain medical services elsewhere.

At that time hospital management corporations were developing rapidly. Portraying themselves as having the practical and technical know-how sorely lacking in the nonprofit sector, they began to acquire and manage hospitals as early as 1968. In the seventies, the management industry experienced a remarkable growth.[11] In 1975 there were 91 privately managed hospitals, with a total of 10,785 beds. In 1976, this increased to 127 hospitals with 16,063 beds. By mid-1977 the Federation of American Hospitals directory reported 202 managed hospitals with a total of 24,181 beds.

NME is a gigantic medical corporation.[12] It was incorporated in 1975 and owns or operates acute, rehabilitative, psychiatric, substance abuse, and long-term facilities in the United States and overseas. In 1989 its total sales amounted to over $3.5 billion, and licensed beds in its chain aggregate 57,557—7,669 in specialty hospitals, 6,726 in general hospitals, and 43,162 in nursing homes. The company is the third largest for-profit health care company in the nation after Hospital Corporation of America and Humana.

Hyatt Corporation is also a mammoth enterprise.[13] Its hotel and other conglomerate operations expanded recently to include the American Medical International, the country's fourth largest hospital company.

The Study Begins

API agreed to study the figures presented by the hospital management firms and the work commenced. Three volunteers were assigned to the case by API: Ronald Born, J. Peter Singer, and myself as supervisor.

Ronald Born, then retired, had had a long career as statistician, budget analyst, and eventually general manager of the Department of Social Services of the City and County of San Francisco. J. Peter Singer was the manager of management services of a leading firm of certified public accountants, and had designed and implemented new accounting systems and improved data processing services in a number of California hospitals.

NME and Hyatt both submitted proposals to provide hospital management services to VMC, and the staff of VMC also submitted its proposal for continued public management. A summary of the cost proposals by the two management firms was as follows:

NME proposed a management fee of $350,000 per year with an annual review based on the work program performed. For this, they proposed the provision of four full-time staff persons, augmented by six full-time equivalent positions from their own organization.

Hyatt proposed a fee of $395,000 per year, with a three-year contract, which included an annual cost of living increase. This fee includes the cost of a hospital administrator. If, however, the county continued to employ the existing administrator and pay his salary and fringe benefits, Hyatt would reduce its annual fee to approximately $345,000.

Before proceeding further with this case study, it is essential to understand why Fresno solicited proposals from management firms in the first place. Both Fresno County and Merced County, which is about 50 miles north of it, are situated in the San Joaquin Valley, one of the most fertile agricultural areas in the world. In 1973, the Merced Community Medical Center (Merced) signed a hospital management contract with NME.

An updated report by NME has the following title:
Merced Community Medical Center
    1973–1974 Review
    1974–1975 Report
    1975–1976 Proposal.

On page 1, item 1, *Financial Performance,* there is the following statement:

The hospital not only lived within the cash flow, but *experienced a $320,000 turnaround* from a negative operational income of $146,000 to a *positive operational income of $180,000* at fiscal year-end. The year-to-date deficit on October 31, 1973, was $146,406 with a $36,601 deficit per month from July 1, 1973 to October 31, 1973. This deficit had been reduced to $28,259 by the end of March due to positive operational income figures of $118,147 from Nov. 1, 1973, through March 31, 1974. By June 30, 1974, a positive operational view of $180,000 had been realized. The prior fiscal year loss had been approximately $500,000. [Underlined in the original.]

In the introduction to this report, NME stated:

Within 12 months after initiation of the service contract, the hospital had a positive accrual of $180,000, and within two years of $462,000. Not only has the turnaround been remarkable, but the positive accrual has been used for the betterment of the hospital.

From an accounting point of view, there is some lack of clarity as to exactly what is supposed to have happened. There is, however, a clear implication that substantial savings were effected during the first year of NME's management of Merced Community Medical Center. On May 12, 1976, the 1975–1976 grand jury of Fresno, California, stated that after a thorough investigation of Valley Medical Center, it was "distressed over the financial burden it [VMC] continues to place on county taxpayers." After repeating, almost verbatim, the two NME quotations above, the grand jury then said that if this management service should be chosen by Fresno County, it estimated that a saving of $5 million to $7 million annually would be realized without any reduction of present services. *The grand jury report does not give the basis for the estimated $5 to $7 million in savings per annum.* The grand jury concluded by urging the Fresno County Board of Supervisors to take immediate action to study the proposals of NME or "any other corporation." On the basis of these representations, the Fresno Board of Supervisors decided to solicit bids from NME and other management firms.

It was obvious to API personnel that, in view of this history, in order to evaluate the bid proposal by NME, it would be necessary to evaluate NME's performance at Merced. On February 23 and 24, 1977, the three API volunteers visited Merced Hospital, VMC and the office of the county administrator in Fresno. On February 23 we conferred with C. Gregg McKown, administrator of Merced Hospital (employed by NME); Clark G. Charming, county administrator of Merced County; and Leroy G. Gilsdorf, auditor, controller, and recorder of Merced County. At the conference we learned about the structure, size and operations of the hospital. The information is summarized in the report issued by API (discussed later in the chapter). When we asked about the claim that NME management had saved about $500,000, none of the hospital and county personnel could confirm or deny it.

On February 24 we visited VMC, where we met with a number of VMC supervising personnel. Here again we accumulated the data describing the hospital operations. On February 24 we also visited Robert A. Butler, the Fresno County administrative officer, who told us of the negotiations with hospital management firms.

Subsequent to these visits, API received copies of the proposals from both NME and Hyatt. In addition, the staff of VMC submitted a proposal of its own, applying for continued county management of the hospital. All of these were accompanied by a number of financial statements and other analytical and statistical data.

Hyatt in its proposal mentioned that it had a management contract with Southern Nevada Memorial Hospital (SNH). The proposal went on to say (and we quote):

> The hospital managed by Hyatt that most closely resembles Valley Medical Center is Southern Nevada Memorial Hospital. It contains in excess of 300 beds and has an annual budget of approximately 29 million dollars. Southern Nevada Memorial Hospital is a multidisciplined teaching hospital serving a patient market area that includes the southern half of the State of Nevada, areas of Northwestern Arizona and Eastern California. This hospital maintains clinical relationships with three medical schools and has rotating residency programs in seven areas.

In its proposal Hyatt also included Exhibit No. 5, a report to Southern Nevada Memorial Hospital (SNH), dated June 29, 1976. Page 2 of the report states that for the year 1975–76, the first year of Hyatt's management, there was an approximate net operating surplus of $500,000 as compared with $1,000,000 deficits in each of the two preceding years. What caused this reported change is not explained in the report. Because of these claims, SNH became an integral part of the study, so that API decided to visit it. On June 17, 1977, my wife (not a member of API) and I did visit the hospital. API's report summarized the data we accumulated. As in the case of Merced, no one was able to confirm or deny the huge reported savings effected by Hyatt. API had gathered a great deal of financial data by this time, not only that provided by the two hospital management firms and the hospital itself, but also other reports it considered to be helpful.

On July 27, 1977, API issued its draft report on the VMC. As was customary, this was reviewed by API's Case Committee, and changes made after thorough discussion and before issuance to the following:

William Plumb of Community Coalition on VMC
API Volunteers: Ronald Born
                    Esmond Coleman
                    Peter Singer
                    Nancy Snodden

Fresno County Board of Supervisors, c/o Robert Butler
 Fresno Grand Jury
 Valley Medical Center, c/o Manuel Perez
 National Medical Enterprises, Inc., c/o Paul F. Avard, Sr.
 VP
 Hyatt Medical Enterprises, Inc./Hyatt Medical
 Management Services, Inc., c/o Dennis Solari
 Hyatt Medical Enterprises, Joaquin Acosta
 Ann Klinger, c/o Merced Board of Supervisors
 Merced Community Medical Center,
  C. Gregg McKown, Administrator
 George Riesz, Administrator,
  Southern Nevada Memorial Hospital

The draft report was accompanied by a letter dated July 27, 1977, asking the recipients to respond in writing to reach API on or before August 5, 1977. It stated that API would consider all such comments and would issue its final report on August 15, 1977. API also asked all the recipients to treat the draft as confidential material because of the sensitivity of the matter. Although it was standard operating procedure for API to request comments from interested parties before issuance of final reports, it was not always necessary to stress the confidentiality of the material. Some of the recipients did respond; others did not. API personnel reviewed the comments and amended the report where they considered it necessary. Once again the report was reviewed by the Case Committee and the final report was issued on August 26, 1977.

The more important aspects of the report are discussed below.

The first and most obvious question to consider was cost savings, because this was the primary reason the Grand Jury of Fresno had recommended that the Board of Supervisors investigate the possibility of contracting with a hospital management firm and that is why the board was doing it.

The reader will recall that NME had claimed that there had been a saving of more than $500,000 during the first year it managed Merced. Since this had not been proven to API personnel by either examination of financial material or interviews with Merced and NME people, API referred to the management of NME.

In a letter to API dated May 6, 1977, Leland R. Cannon, vice president, Management Services of NME, stated:

You state specifically you are interested in verifying the savings which NME claimed were effected in the first fiscal year of management. I have personally heard statements outside the confines of my company and in varying amounts, that such claims were made. I have no knowledge of the accuracy of these contentions, but can only refer to the published statements and the results reflected therein.

This is an interesting letter because *the source of the claim was the report published by NME itself.*

In its first audit report for Merced, years ended June 30, 1976 and 1975, Hurdman and Cranstoun, Certified Public Accountants, stated on page 10, note 6:

Restated financial statements for the fiscal year ended June 30, 1974, have not been presented since financial statements were not issued or prepared for that year.

If this was the first year of NME's management of Merced, it is clear that there could be no valid claim for savings. So much for NME's savings.

It will also be recalled that Hyatt, in its proposal to VMC and in publicity generally, had claimed very substantial savings for SNH during the first two years of its management of that Nevada facility. We asked George Riesz, administrator of SNH, Ron Trace, vice president of Hyatt, and Dennis Solari, hospital group controller of Hyatt what evidence they could produce substantiating such savings. The answer was *none.*

Although in these two cases, savings were not proved, it should be emphasized that there may appear to be savings when in fact there are none, or they may be exaggerated. Let us consider how this may happen.

Traditionally, county hospitals were not operated as independent business entities. Because the county was legally obligated to treat indigent patients, for example, the county hospital would do so and bill neither the indigent patient nor the county, since the patient could not pay, and there seemed to be no point in billing the county. After all, if the hospital did not get paid for such services it would get paid by the county at the end of the year on a lump-sum deficit basis or during the year with funds as needed by the hospital to make up deficits. That bothers everybody. The board of supervisors points to county hospital losses accusingly. Taxpayers grumble at the board and the hospital administrator and say, "Throw the rascals out!" The hospital administrator gets humble and beats his breast, promising to do better in the future, or he gets defiant and abusive.

Suppose now a hospital management firm comes in and changes the game plan. The hospital bills the county for service to indigents, collects from the county on a current basis, and needs less end-of-the-year or deficit financing from the county. Superficially it looks as if the hospital is doing better financially, or to put it differently, it has effected savings, reduced its deficit, made a turnaround, etc.

Actually, nothing has been changed except the way in which the county pays the same amount of money to the county hospital.

Basically, this book does not attempt to evaluate the quality of health service made available to the indigent. However, where a hospital firm claims that it has saved or will save money, one must look at how that has been or will be accomplished. This question is explored in a report to the National Health Law Program by Ruth Roemer, J.D., entitled "Administration of County General Hospitals in California by Private Management Firms," August 9, 1977. The report points out, for example, that the elimination of outpatient clinics and the substitution of emergency clinics may save money, but "emergency room care is well known to be episodic and discontinuous care, with no preventive services, little follow-up, and minimal monitoring or quality control."

In the case of county hospitals a comparison of operations for different years may be difficult, if not impossible, because of changing accounting methods. Because the county had the responsibility to provide medical service to its inhabitants, the county hospital was regarded not as a free-standing organization but as one of the arms of county administration. It was usually run on a cash basis rather than on an accrual basis, even though its expenses and revenues were readily susceptible to accrual. That is, the expenses could be recorded when incurred rather than when paid and its revenues could be recorded when billed rather than when received. The accrual basis of accounting and the treatment of a county hospital as a free-standing financial unit is known as the enterprise fund system. It includes an overhauling of the billing system, so that, like other independent hospitals, whether nonprofit or proprietary, all billings should be recorded at full price, and allowances and bad debts of all kinds should be segregated as reductions of revenue. Unquestionably, this is far superior to the prior method and offers a measure of control over operations that was not available under the old system. However, it does not necessarily follow that if the first year of the enterprise fund system shows a smaller loss than the previous year of the cash basis system, savings were effected. Such a conclusion would only be correct if proven after a thorough analysis of the figures involved. It might even be impossible for lack of comparable data for the two years.

One avenue of possible saving to a county hospital is a more aggressive and stringent policy of collecting hospital bills by litigation with the possible result that indigent people in need of medical care are discouraged from seeking admission to the hospital. As has been mentioned, Fresno is in the heart of San Joaquin Valley, a very fertile agricultural area. Large numbers of undocumented Mexican nationals are in demand by the so-called factories in the field. They and a number of other poor people are at risk if a very stringent policy of hospital access is instituted, because they fear they might be deported if they cannot pay their hospital bills.

As has been mentioned, a matter of serious concern to those interested in the welfare of the hospital was the experience any of the hospital management firms had had in the administration of a so-called teaching hospital, or a hospital of the size of VMC. The following table shows a comparison of VMC, Merced (the comparable hospital cited by NME), and SNH (the comparable facility cited by Hyatt):

	VMC[14]	MERCED[15]	SNH[16]
Number of beds	364	124	205
Occupancy rate	76%	68.5%	NA
Occupied beds	276.5	85	NA
Teaching history	70 yrs.	minor	minor

It is apparent that there is limited comparability as to size between Merced, SNH, and VMC, and no comparability at all as to the teaching function.

In the state of California it is required that each hospital submit a very detailed statistical and financial report on its operations each year to the California Health Facilities Commission. As these reports are available to the public and are uniform in format, it is not very difficult to compare various operations of one hospital with others. API made a number of such comparisons; the functions compared included fee collection efficiency, financial management procedures, variances in department costs, cost containment, overstaffing, unit costs, etc. Although there were great differences between VMC statistics as compared to the same statistics of the county hospitals in Kings, Madera, Mariposa, Merced, and Tulare (all in California), no overall conclusion could be drawn as to superiority or inferiority; all were better in some ways and worse in others.

In spite of determined efforts to do so, API was unable to ascertain the names and qualifications of managers each of the management firms proposed to place in VMC.

Taking all of the factors above into account, API concluded that there was insufficient evidence that Fresno County would derive any greater benefit from the use of an outside management firm than from the continuation of county management. We reached this conclusion by asking why Fresno County should engage a facility manager. If the reason is to reduce costs, we found no evidence in the other hospitals visited to suggest that contract management alone results in reduced costs. In the case of both of the hospitals cited as examples of what could be achieved, there was no documentation of savings. We concluded that the improved financial stability reported at both of the managed hospitals was a mirage created by changed accounting procedures. We also concluded that prior management of both managed hospitals was less effective than the present management of VMC. If the reason was better management, then Fresno County is entitled to know who the managers would be so they could judge the relative merits of the individuals. As a corollary, we also believe the county should be more able to identify specific deficiencies of present management. If the reason is better systems and procedures, Fresno should contract specifically for these improvements.

At the same time, however, we also concluded that if present management is retained, or new resident management is chosen, it can, in our judgment, be successful only if:

A. The board of supervisors will be more directly involved as the board of the hospital. We were impressed with the arrangement in Merced County in which the board meets regularly as the board of the hospital. We understand that a similar arrangement is in effect in Clark County (Southern Nevada Hospital). They meet at the hospital with no other items on their agenda. By so doing, the board can be more directly involved in setting policy and in overseeing the effectiveness of hospital management.

B. The board of supervisors will set realistic goals for hospital management and force management to report against those goals. If the goals are not met, then the board can determine whether to replace the management of the hospital.

C. The board of supervisors establishes a salary structure and/or working conditions for the position of chief financial officer that will enable VMC to attract and *retain* a competent financial manager. We understand that this position has been occupied by no fewer than three individuals in the past three to four years. Further, additional positions in the financial department may be required for budgeting and financial analysis and for expertise in government reimbursement.

D. The county retains consultant services to: develop and *implement* a management reporting system; clean out the old accounts receivable and establish an effective credit and collections procedure; improve the pricing structure to maximize reimbursement; define and select an appropriate data processing vendor and oversee the system implementation; assist in further improving or formalizing the cost containment program already established. Some or all of these services may be offered by NME, Hyatt, or other hospital management firms; by a large CPA firm; or by a hospital consultant firm. We believe that dollars spent on specific projects to augment county management can be at least as effective as hiring a firm for overall management.

E. The resident managership is given adequate responsibility and authority to function and expend funds in accordance with policy established in A through D above, without crippling limitations. We have noted that, all too frequently, a facility manager is given resources and authority not previously accorded county management.

On August 26, 1977, API issued its report, which was substantially the same as the draft report issued to all concerned parties on July 27, 1977. The final report took into consideration comments received from those commenting on the draft report. On August 29, 1977, the Fresno County Board of Supervisors held a public meeting at which VMC, Hyatt and NME presented their proposals. The printed announcement of the meeting stated that there would be presentations or comments by interested groups and members of the public, including:

Valley Medical Center Advisory Board
    Community Coalition on Valley Medical Center
    Accountants for the Public Interest

VMC Medical Staff
Fresno County Grand Jury
County Administrative Officer

In addition to these, others made comments. The discussion was spirited and indeed at times acrimonious. No vote was taken at the time, but subsequently, the board of supervisors voted three to two to retain county management for the time being.

One More Time

It seemed at the time that the problem had been disposed of, but such was not the case. In November, 1983, the community coalition again asked API to assist them in analyzing some financial projection documents presented to the Fresno County Board of Supervisors by County Administrative Officer Allan Coleman, to justify the tremendous savings to be realized by the county upon the transfer of ownership and control of VMC to a private, nonprofit entity. The memorandum dated November 7, 1983, is so amazing that I cannot refrain from reporting a summary of the first two pages:

Date: November 7, 1983
To: Board of Supervisors
From: Allan H. Coleman, CAO
Subject: Valley Medical Center

We have now completed the first detailed financial projections concerning the County continuing to operate Valley Medical Center versus a nonprofit corporation. Fresno County would save an estimated $44,900,000 over the next 10 years if a nonprofit corporation operated VMC. Of equal significance is that the nonprofit corporation would be able to generate an estimated $67.4 million in debt capacity with which they could fund expansion and improvement of the entire medical center. Based upon the just completed Price Waterhouse audit of VMC for 1982–83, and assuming that patient census, inflation projections, and reimbursement programs remain stable, we believe the $44,900,000 figure is conservative. With reference to the development of debt capacity, one of the most significant issues we have had with the VMC budget the last few years is our inability to raise funds to improve and expand VMC. At the end of the first year of operation of a nonprofit corporation, $22.8 million worth of debt capacity for expansion purposes should already be achievable.

The letter then presents figures I am summarizing as follows:

Valley Medical Center
Nonprofit vs. County Operated Estimate of
Ten-Year Projects
(000's)

	Net county cost 1984–1993 inclusive
County operated	$135,600
Nonprofit operated	90,700
Cost savings to county	$44,900

What makes it so amazing is that without a shred of proof to justify the saving of one two-cent postage stamp, the CAO offers this document to explain the saving of $45 million in 10 years, if the ownership of the VMC is transferred to a nonprofit entity (consisting of the doctors currently working at VMC). The memorandum on November 14, 1983, repeats some of the same statements about projected savings and calls for a public hearing on November 28, 1983. In a telephone conversation with the coalition spokesman prior to the November 28 hearing, I listed a number of financial documents that would be required to make an informed decision and stated that if these or similar materials were not provided to the public, the legislative procedure should be considered completely inadequate and should be so characterized. Subsequently, I was informed that at the public hearing, accounting personnel of VMC came forward with figures proving that the continuation of county operation would be far more advantageous than leasing the county hospital to a nonprofit organization. The matter has been shelved for the time being.

Unfortunately, as in the case of the excision of a cancerous growth, one is never sure of the eventual result. Will metastasis set in, and if so, when and where?

. The Broader Picture

The case of VMC indicates clearly that in this case it was not advantageous to transfer the management of the hospital to a management firm, but it also served to institute a more extensive study of private management of seven public hospitals in California by William Shonick, Ph.D., and Ruth Roemer, J.D., of the School of Public Health, University of California, Los Angeles. They contracted with me and Van Keulen and Lumer, CPAs, to consult on the fiscal aspects of the study. The seven hospitals selected for study were Harold B. Chope Community Hospital (San Mateo County), Highland General Hospital (Alameda County), Mendocino Community Hospital, Merced Community Medical Center, Community Hospital of Sonoma County, Santa Clara Valley Medical Center, and Sutter Community Hospital. All of them had been managed by private hospital management firms for part or all of the years from 1973 to 1980.

As explained previously, in the state of California, all hospitals were then required by law to submit an annual comprehensive financial and statistical report to the California Health Facilities Commission (C.H.F.C.). For the purpose of this study, it was agreed that these reports were to be analyzed, since being uniform for all hospitals they offered a good resource for analysis of the financial experience in the years of private management for each hospital. In addition, audited financial statements, when available, were examined, and we also visited facilities.

The study by Dr. Shonick and Dr. Roemer was published by the Institute of Governmental Studies of the University of California, Berkeley, in 1983 under the title *Public Hospitals Under Private Management—The California Experience*. The authors were concerned with the following key questions:

1. Does private management reduce net county costs?
2. Does private management overcome the constraints of county government?
3. Does private management restrict patient access?
4. Does private management affect the quality of care?
5. Does private management diminish public accountability?

The findings concerning questions 1 and 5 may be briefly summarized as follows.

Examining the obligations and problems faced by public hospitals in both rural and urban areas of California, the researchers found that no cost savings or savings to the county were achieved that were attributable to more efficient management in any of the hospitals studied. The one county hospital where savings to the county were achieved (but not overall savings) occurred because of cross-subsidization, that is, transferring some of the cost of county patients to private insurers, especially Blue Cross, through higher charges for privately insured patients.

On the issue of public accountability, the evidence was mixed. In two counties, where the board of supervisors were eager to be relieved of hospital problems, the management firm served to distance the board from the hospital and the public. In other counties where the board remained quite involved in hospital affairs, there was still some concern about "dual allegiance" of the administrator to the management firm and to the county, but no hard evidence indicated that the administrator's allegiance created administrative difficulties.

In looking at future trends, the authors expressed the following fundamental policy concern:

We consider the continuing consolidation of these chains to be a fundamental public policy concern, with the prospect of a future in which public hospitals become part of huge, for-profit corporate hospital chains that dominate the field, in the way the "seven sisters" dominate the oil industry. What will be the prospects for changes the public may want to make in the health system, if the system, including public hospitals, is owned and/or operated by an oligopoly of huge corporate chains? What will government have to pay to such monopolies to serve the public need?

Beyond Acute Care Hospitals

We are not ready to leave the subject of hospital management firms. On February 11, 1983, an article entitled "Mill Valley Uproar over Convalescent Center," by Richard R. Leger, appeared in the *San Francisco Chronicle*. It concerns Hillhaven Convalescent Center in Marin County, California. The center was operated by NME, one of the hospital management firms I discussed in the Fresno County Hospital case. The article stated that the convalescent center, the third largest in Marin County, was closing its doors and that its 110 patients would have to move out within two months. The old people and their relatives, some in great distress, were forced to hurriedly compete with each other for new beds in a region where such space is desperately scarce.

The operators intended to convert the facility into a low-overhead type of alcohol and drug treatment center. To accomplish this, special legislation was introduced in the state legislature on September 11, 1981, and was passed and signed into law within 15 days. The legislation was introduced at the request of NME, enabling it to avoid the normal hearing process to qualify for a "certificate of need" from the state to make the conversion from convalescent home to drug rehabilitation center. It sent a formal application for the conversion to Sacramento. On June 3 it received the state "certificate of need" that permits the conversion subject to other necessary licenses. It lined up medical directors to run the new operation that will replace the nursing home. Hillhaven patients weren't warned of the impending closing of the nursing home because it might have hurt business, according to the operators. Advance notice "was considered, but if you hint to somebody it might be closed and isn't, you're setting up a facility for failure," said Robert Peirce, Northern California director of operations for Hillhaven, which operates 49 nursing homes in California and 270 in the United States as a subsidiary of NME.

This was NME's plan, but it did not work out that way. NME was unable to get the license to convert the convalescent home as planned, and the facility is still (1991) a convalescent home.

When one considers the case of VMC, the study of California hospital management firms and the Hillhaven Convalescent Home incident, one is forced to conclude with Paul Starr when he wrote that "corporations have begun to integrate a hitherto decentralized hospital system, enter a variety of health care businesses, and consolidate ownership and control in what may eventually become an industry dominated by huge health care conglomerates."[17]

In that world the name of the game is not health, but money, and the hospital management firms are among the leaders.

3. Nursing Homes—San Francisco and Berkeley, California

In acute care or general hospitals we have been describing thus far, the average length of stay is between six and seven days. In nursing homes the vast majority of residents remain from the date of admission until death, or until they are evicted because of financial insolvency.

The general term "nursing homes" will be used in this discussion to include long-term care facilities with various names such as skilled nursing facilities, convalescent homes, intermediate care facilities, nursing homes, guest homes, foster homes, group homes, board and care homes, etc. In order to understand how nursing homes deny care to many indigent people it is necessary to understand some salient characteristics of the industry.

Because the San Francisco nursing home study, which is one of the subjects of this chapter, was performed in the late 1970s, most of the statistics quoted hereafter relate to that period; occasionally more recent figures are cited for comparison purposes.

There is a profound difference between the ages of patients in acute care hospitals and in nursing homes. In acute care hospitals, ages of patients range from infancy to old age. In nursing homes the ages of patients are in the higher age brackets. In 1977 and 1985, if we ignore the residents under 65, and they were relatively few, the resident age groups were as follows:[1]

| | 1977 | | 1985 | |
| | Residents | | Residents | |
Age	in thousands	%	in thousands	%
65–74	211	19%	212	16%
75–84	465	41%	509	39%
85 and over	450	40%	597	45%
Total	1,126	100%	1,318	100%

The increasing percentage of the 85 and older group from 40% to 45% presents the system with severe social and financial problems. Medicaid assumes much of the burden, which might be alleviated to a large extent if home care services (discussed later in this book) were utilized more effectively.

The growth of the nursing home business has been phenomenal in recent years—total annual expenditures on nursing home care rose from $4.2 billion in 1964 to $34.7 in 1985 after adjustment for inflation.[2]

An indication of the extent to which nursing homes are involved with the indigent can be understood when we realize that in 1981, of total Medicaid expenses of $29.7 billion, 40.3%, or $12 billion, went to nursing homes.

Nursing homes in the United States are primarily privately owned. In 1978, for example, according to Table No. 171 of the *1982–83 Statistical Abstract of the United States,* a comparison of nursing homes and general hospitals is as follows:

	Nursing Homes	%	Hospitals	%
Under Government Control	1,214	7%	2,607	36%
Under Profit Control	14,023	74%	958	13%
Under Nonprofit Control	3,485	19%	3,594	51%
Total	18,722	100%	7,159	100%

Private nonprofit institutions, tax-exempt as most are under Section 501(c)(3) of the Internal Revenue Code, rely heavily on contributions from individuals who claim them as tax deductions. This source of revenue is not available to institutions operating for profit. Consequently, most nursing homes must rely on revenue received from residents and Medicaid, with a small amount coming from Medicare.

With these facts in mind we can proceed to our case study.

In 1976 the Community Coalition for Nursing Home Reform (San Francisco), consisting of the American Jewish Congress, Western Gerontological Society, the San Francisco Department of Social Services and a number of other health professional and consumer groups, requested that Accountants for the Public Interest (API) conduct a financial study of nursing homes in San Francisco County. The purpose of the study was to determine the average cost of providing nursing home care in the county, the adequacy of the Medicaid (Medi-Cal in California) reimbursement rate to cover these costs, and sources of revenues received by these facilities.

The concern of the coalition had been triggered by the fact that on June 4, 1975, 12 San Francisco nursing homes announced that they would no longer accept new Medi-Cal patients and would discharge existing Medi-Cal patients because current costs were not being covered by the state's reimbursement rate.[3] Legal action by a public interest law firm prevented this concerted effort from succeeding. Nonetheless, the proportion of Medi-Cal patients admitted to individual homes began to drop. By 1976 the proportion of Medi-Cal patients in San Francisco homes had dropped to less than 22% of the total patient population, compared to 60% in 1974.

API accepted the case. The financial analysis was performed by Emilio Gonzalez with the assistance of about 20 volunteers and the guidance of a steering committee consisting of myself and two other certified public accountants, Marilyn Johnson and Sara Moore.

Normally a health facility regards an investigative body like API as a combination of the FBI, CIA, and IRS, intent upon locking its head and hands in the pillory. Information is supplied reluctantly, if at all. In this case, however, the situation was quite different. Hoping that the result of API's investigation might result in an increase of fees, the nursing homes cooperated enthusiastically. They gave us copies of financial statements, Medi-Cal cost reports, statistics, etc.

While conducting the study, members of API visited practically all of the nursing homes in San Francisco, always with advance notice, so that things looked shipshape when we arrived.

The data was analyzed thoroughly and a lengthy report, complete with descriptions, tables, and graphs was issued. Basically, the report was limited in scope to the concerns expressed by the community coalition. To understand the nursing home problem more fully it is necessary to discuss certain factors alluded to briefly or not at all in the report.

For many years, the scandal of nursing home care has been exhaustively studied. I shall mention here a few of those studies:

Tender Loving Greed by Mary Adelaide Mendelson, Alfred A. Knopf, 1974

Too Old, Too Sick, Too Bad by Frank E. Moss and Val J. Halamandaris, Aspen Systems Corporation, 1977

Unloving Care by Bruce C. Vladeck, Basic Books, Inc. Publishers, 1980

All these books express outrage at the deplorable conditions in the nursing homes. That will be covered in another section of this book.

Another topic not discussed here is the method of governmental supervision of nursing homes. That consists of the last refuge of a bureaucrat—conduct a survey. There have been countless surveys but nothing changes.

API's report summarized its findings as follows:

1. The average cost per patient per day for skilled nursing services in San Francisco over the past three years is $25.62.
2. The Medi-Cal reimbursement rate is not high enough to cover these costs. It hasn't been adequate for the past three years, and the gap is widening.
3. Last year 54% of San Francisco's Medi-Cal placements were in nursing homes in other counties, and the number of aged poor being served is declining at an accelerating rate.
4. San Francisco nursing homes are increasingly serving the private patient who can afford to pay the higher rates, which currently run $34.50 per day, on the average, for a double room. The present Medi-Cal reimbursement rate is $22.53 per day for a 100-bed facility.
5. Those homes that accept Medi-Cal in payment spend less per day on direct patient care, and more on administration, than do those facilities serving the private-pay patient.
6. Facility costs and nursing salaries lead the way in making San Francisco the highest cost area in the state.
7. Overall, revenues averaged $25.64 per patient day; one third from Medi-Cal, 56% from private sources, 8% from Medicare, and 3% for ancillary and other services.
8. The above figures relate to the period 1974–1976.

These conclusions are clear but they lead to several other observations. One is that the state of California while Ronald Reagan was governor had systematically set about to hamstring Medi-Cal, the primary source of funds to pay for health services for the indigent. Reagan in 1970 appointed Dr. Earl Brian, Jr., a young flight surgeon, to the position of head of the Medi-Cal program. Dr. Brian almost immediately instituted a cumbersome system of Medi-Cal reporting that discouraged and hampered reimbursement.

He also set up a "Schedule of Maximum Allowances," establishing dollar limits on payments for Medi-Cal reimbursement, including payments to nursing homes. Some time later I visited Sacramento to attempt to find out how the maximum allowance rate had been established in this case, for home health agencies. I was told that the man responsible for setting the rate had died. After offering my condolences, I explained that I was interested not in the man, but in the method. I never found out who set the rates or how.

Another thing that is clear from an examination of the report is that the nursing homes were primarily concerned, as profit-making entities, with the making of profits. If this was in conflict with the health needs of the residents, that was regrettable but unavoidable. As a matter of cold fact, sending an elderly nursing home resident to a strange community removes him or her from friends and relatives, and can be, and frequently is, a death sentence. It is usually described as transfer trauma.

An indication of the extent to which government policy and the nursing home industry denied service to the indigent of San Francisco may be illustrated by the following simple statistics of Medi-Cal revenue as a percentage of the nursing home revenue:

For California state-wide	1979–1980	64%
For San Francisco	1979–1980	47%

Nursing homes have some difficulty in getting adequate reimbursement for Medi-Cal services rendered. Acute care hospitals do not have that problem to the same extent. That is because they are controlled by physicians and hospitals. They are very well organized, with powerful professional organizations and a great deal of money available to exert political clout. Nursing homes, on the other hand, are usually controlled by nurses with considerably less influence.

However, this is not a great problem for the nursing homes. With the marked increase in the number of elderly people in our society, the demand for nursing home beds in many cases exceeds the supply, so that nursing homes are frequently in the enviable position, from an economic point of view, if not a humane one, of picking and choosing patients. Consequently, if the Medi-Cal reimbursement rate is low, the Medi-Cal patients can be dropped.

The *Financial Study of Skilled Nursing Facilities* was published by API on November 29, 1977. It covered the period from 1974 to 1976, and made several recommendations, the first two, and the most important of which, were:

1. That the state (California) adjust the Medi-Cal reimbursement rate to cover reasonable costs and provide for a reasonable rate of return as set forth in the Social Security Act.
2. That the state establish a rate differential, by geographic region, to allow for varying costs of providing nursing care in different areas of the state.

On October 15, 1979, the California Department of Consumer Affairs, Board of Medical Quality Assurance, issued a report referring to API's financial study, and recommended the support of the two recommendations. Consequent changes were made.

The Aftermath

Eleven years later, in July, 1990, I called most of the nursing homes in San Francisco and asked them if they had any space available for Medi-Cal patients. In all cases the answer was that no beds were available at this time and they did not know when any would be.

When my wife called the same nursing homes to inquire whether beds were available for full-pay patients the response was somewhat different. In one case a bed was available, and in the others they expected to have vacancies soon. Instead of giving the cursory "no," to me, they stated that they welcomed tours of the premises, offered to send brochures, mentioned recreational facilities and occupational therapies, and assured her that ample parking space was available.

An explanation of the two varying reactions may be found in the fact that the Medi-Cal rate was about $67 per day for skilled nursing care and about $45 for intermediate care whereas the rates for full-pay patients ranged from $88 to $200 per day.[4]

As mentioned earlier, the California Department of Consumer Affairs did agree to adjust the geographic rate structure and in the case of San Francisco, the Medi-Cal rate increased from $26 per day in 1974–76 to about twice that rate in 1990. One might conclude, therefore, that API's report succeeded in its purpose.

But the real question, as always, is where did the money go? The potential Medi-Cal patients are *still* not admitted to nursing homes, or at best, minimally. *The money went to the nursing home proprietors.*

We may conclude this case by quoting from *The Battle of Blenheim,* a poem written by Robert Southey in 1798. In it an old man is telling his two grandchildren about the battle that laid waste the land far and wide and killed thousands of people. At the end of the poem the following colloquy takes place between the grandfather and his grandson:

> "But what good came of it at last?"
> Quoth little Peterkin.
> "Why that I cannot tell," said he,
> "But 'twas a famous victory."

The Berkeley Alta Bates Nursing Home Experience

In 1981, United Neighbors in Action (UNA), a nonprofit organization serving as advocates for the elderly and disabled in Northern California, approached Van Keulen & Lumer (VK&L), a certified public accounting firm with which I was associated. In brief, UNA was concerned with the performance of nursing homes controlled by the Alta Bates Corporation.

Without attempting to discuss in detail the elaborate corporate structure of the Alta Bates Hospital and its related entities, we must understand certain of the ramifications.

The Alta Bates Corporation was established in 1981 to coordinate the health care providing entities controlled by Alta Bates Hospital. These included the 317-bed hospital in Berkeley, California, the 39-bed hospital in Albany, California, Alta Bates Ambulatory Health Services, Inc., which administered sports medicine, home health, hospice and commercial laboratory programs, Alta Bates Foundation, and the Guardian Skilled Nursing Facilities Foundation.

This foundation, according to its Articles of Incorporation filed in the Office of the Secretary of State of California in 1975, was formed for the following reason:

> The specific and primary purposes are to acquire, own and operate Skilled Nursing Facilities, as defined in the Medicare Act, 42 USC 1395X(j), to receive and maintain gifts of money and property to Alta Bates Hospital or for charitable, scientific and educational activities related to Alta Bates Hospital.

The CT-2 filing with the Attorney General of California states that the "Organization provides skilled nursing services in its operation of convalescent hospitals."

The Guardian Foundation owns and manages seven convalescent

hospitals, ranging in size from 36 to 155 available beds.

The fundamental question posed by UNA was: Do the Alta Bates Convalescent Hospitals meet the needs of the community? Our accounting firm agreed that we would proceed with the analysis of annual reports submitted to the Attorney General of California, Form CT-2 required of nonprofit organizations (all of the related entities were nonprofit) and annual reports that must be submitted by all nursing homes to the California Health Facilities Commission. The legal and accounting complexities of all the Alta Bates entities are not the subject of this study. What I shall describe is the operations of the Alta Bates nursing homes. The following tabulation comes from the California Health Facilities Commission:[5]

	PATIENT DAYS		**CHARGE PER DAY**	
	7	**1110**	**7**	**1110**
	Alta Bates Homes	**Statewide Homes**	**Alta Bates Homes**	**Statewide Homes**
Medicare	5.9%	2.5%	$26.67	$37.33
Medicaid (Medi-Cal)	11.0%	69.6%	24.21	29.58
Private	83.0%	27.2%	43.23	38.27
Other	.1%	.7%	36.25	37.78
Total	100.0%	100.0%	$40.13	$32.20

From this tabulation it is obvious how and why the Alta Bates convalescent homes fared so well financially. Their private-pay residents with the highest charge per day, $43.23, constituted 83.0% of their resident population, whereas the statewide heavy caseload was Medi-Cal residents, 69.6%, with the lowest charge, $29.58 per day. To put it bluntly, as in the case of the proprietary and nonprofit hospitals, those patients who can afford higher fees are preferred to those who cannot.

The Alta Bates Hospital claimed that it was necessary to maximize profits of its nursing homes because the hospital itself was losing money on its Medi-Cal operations, and therefore needed additional revenue.[6] As I mentioned earlier, this is a common complaint by hospitals. It sounds convincing, but it must be examined in the light of what happened in late 1982. The following excerpt comes from the *San Francisco Chronicle,* November 18, 1982:

A drastic shift in where San Francisco's 85,000 Medi-Cal patients will get hospital care starting the first of next year was revealed yesterday. State officials disclosed nine hospitals in the city that have won exclusive Medi-Cal contracts.

Left out are many of the hospitals that historically have served a high percentage of the city's indigent. Experts expect some of these hospitals that lost contracts to close.

Some officials at hospitals that lost out were stunned.

The article went on to say that French Hospital, Mount Zion Hospital, and others complained bitterly that the loss in volume would be disastrous for them. The winners were delighted.

Subsequently, when contracts were awarded in the area occupied by Alta Bates Hospital, Alta Bates was one of those selected. They did not turn down the contract, even though "they were losing money!"

Several obvious conclusions are ignored by the planners of our health care system:

1. The use of home health service instead of nursing homes, whether reimbursed by Medicaid or other insurance, can be less expensive and more humane. (See Chapter 4.)
2. Nursing homes that do not accept Medicaid patients, when no other plan is available, force the indigent into county hospitals, jails or into the ranks of the homeless—cruel and wasteful solutions.
3. The vast majority of American citizens live in dread of being warehoused in nursing homes when they are aged and incapable of caring for themselves completely. They fear the possible inadequate care, the neglect, filthy living conditions, and, because of the constantly mounting costs, bankruptcy of themselves and their families. Above all they feel that the money spent results not in health care, but in the loss of their personalities and self-respect. They are horrified of becoming urine-soaked, bed-sore–ridden derelicts.

4. In-Home Services

Up to now we have considered medical services provided in institutions, but at this point we wish to explore the subject of medical services rendered to patients in their homes. As we shall see, the latter are frequently more appropriate for the patient, the patient's family and the financial cost to them and the community in general. There are three such types of service in this group: home health services, hospice, and AIDS. The last one, AIDS, is so catastrophic and complex it will not be included here but in the following chapter.

Home Health Services

Home health services are health and other supportive services provided to people in their own homes. Sometimes it is regarded as a cheap, second-class substitute for institutional health care. That is a mistaken notion. Under proper conditions it is a more appropriate solution for the individual and his or her family in a variety of important ways. If a person is physically, emotionally, and mentally able to live alone or with a spouse when supported by visiting nurses, physical therapists, occupational therapists, and other specialized therapists and homemaker/home health aides, such a person will probably be happier and more related to reality than if he or she were confined in an institution. Most individuals do not need all of the personnel listed above. In some cases help with shopping, cooking, and housecleaning, under the supervision of a nurse, may be sufficient. Each case has to be judged on its own merits. Usually the services in the home are less costly to the individual and society.

As discussed by Brahna Trager in her book *Homemaker/Home Health Aide Services in the United States,*[1] "home help" programs in European countries are far more advanced in scope, percentage of population helped, and general acceptance as a right rather than a privilege, than they are in the United States. This is true for a number of reasons. The first program in Europe to provide home health services was in Frankfurt, Germany, in 1892, as compared to the United States, where, although it was started in the early part of the 20th century, it did not develop to any marked extent until the middle of the century. And even then, the extent of the program was not nearly as complete as in European countries. For example, in 1958, the United States had 143 agencies with both full-time and part-time employees aggregating 1,715. Finland, in 1957, with a population 2.5% that of the United States, employed over 1,715 workers. A comparison of programs in Sweden, Denmark, Norway, Great Britain, and other European countries displayed similar profiles.

There are several reasons for the differences between the program of the United States and European countries. One important reason is the fact that two wars in European territory caused major family upsets, and a consequent attempt to have trained personnel introduced into family life to support healthy patterns of child care. Another reason was the tighter family structure in Europe, where the home, as the important life center, prevented the extensive development of institutions.

In a report entitled *Reasons for Assistance—Task of the Home Health Agency,* there is an innovative discussion of the attitude of the program in Sweden in 1965.[2] In essence, it states that nobody should stay in an institution if the person's social or medical problems can be solved in other ways. Even the indigent lacking lodging, furniture, or the ability to clothe, clean or cook for himself or herself, can be provided for with lodging, etc., and at the same time be independent. Families should not be broken, but should be counseled and helped wherever possible, if home services are appropriate. This program is not only more humane than institutional care, but far less expensive.

It can also be used to enhance family relationships; my own family is a case in point. When my father-in-law, an elderly widower living alone, found it difficult to perform all the necessary household tasks, we arranged for a homemaker to visit him several times a week, clean his apartment, help him with cooking and shopping, etc. My father-in-law was physically healthy and mentally alert. He felt that the homemaker was not only helpful but also a welcome visitor. In addition, if any problems arose, the home health agency notified us, so that we felt quite secure about his condition. All of this was accomplished at a small fraction of the cost of his being housed in an institution, and with a far greater personal sense of satisfaction and dignity for him.

In the United States, in 1965, Medicare and Medicaid became law and operative in 1966 as federal and state programs, respectively.

These should have resulted in a marked expansion of home health services, but what did happen? Not nearly as much as might have been expected, for reasons that will be elucidated as we proceed. In the first place, as Val J. Halamandaris states, "In 1975, nursing homes received over $5 billion from Medicaid's $15 billion total. As a result of a 1967 amendment offered by Senator Moss, Medicaid authorized payment for home health services. But funding has never reached even one percent of the total program."[3]

In addition, as I know well from my experience as a CPA for one of the largest home health agencies in the country, the regulations established by the U.S. government and its fiscal intermediaries are contradictory and very onerous. The overreliance on institutional care and a search for miracle solutions to the health industry in the United States (let us say "cost containment") further compound the problem.

Before discussing the restrictive nature of the Medicare regulations, it is necessary to discuss home health services in a little more depth. A *home health agency* is a public or private agency that specializes in giving skilled nursing services and other therapeutic services, such as physical therapy, in the home. Usually the service is limited to professional nursing plus another service, such as home health aide service or some other form of therapy. The agency may also provide other supportive services, such as assistance in ambulation and a bath, but frowns upon basic services such as shopping, housekeeping, etc.

A *homemaker agency* basically provides the supportive services without nursing and other forms of therapy.

The home helpers are called *home health aides* in the home health agency, and *homemakers* in the homemaker agencies.

The most important Medicare restriction is that Medicare will pay only for home health agency services, and not for homemaker services.

The January 1983 edition of *Your Medicare Handbook* published by the U.S. Department of Health and Human Services sums it up this way (pages 37 and 38):

If you need part-time skilled health care in your home for the treatment of an illness or injury, Medicare can pay for covered home health visits furnished by a participating home health agency.

Medicare can pay for home health visits only if all of the following four conditions are met: (1) the care you need includes part-time skilled nursing care, physical therapy, or speech therapy, (2) you are confined to your home, (3) a doctor determines you need home health care and sets up a home health plan for you, and (4) the home health agency providing services is participating in Medicare.

Once these conditions are met, either hospital insurance or medical insurance can pay for an unlimited number of home health visits. When you no longer need part-time skilled nursing care, physical therapy, or speech therapy, Medicare does *not* continue to pay for home health visits.

Medicare does *not* cover general household services, meal preparation, shopping, assistance in bathing or dressing, or other home care services furnished mainly to assist people in meeting personal, family, or domestic needs.

In essence, what we are being told here is that Medicare will pay for treatment and cure of illness and disease but not for prevention. At a time when we are deluged by complaints of the high cost of Medicare, there is no understanding, apparently, that cure is far more expensive and far less helpful than prevention. This Medicare restriction, of course, applies to hospital, nursing home and physician services as well as to home care services.

An Alternative Program

In October, 1972, the same year the Senate Special Committee on Aging issued its report urging less restrictive Medicare home health service, P.L. 92-603 was enacted. Also known as the Social Security Amendment of 1972 or H.R.I., Section 222 of this law required that Demonstration Projects be conducted to determine if other levels of less intensive care provided in the community would reduce the utilization of inpatient levels of care and whether these levels would improve the care of patients and at what cost.

The legislation suggested that, in addition to intermediate care, Day Care (or, to use the new term, Adult Day Health Care Services) and Homemaker Services should be provided to test their effectiveness, and to determine whether these levels of care should be incorporated into the package of Medicare benefits.

Several communities in the country were funded to test the cost and patient outcome effectiveness of Adult Day Health Care Services and Homemaker Services. The San Francisco Project was the largest and began operations in May, 1975. The project ended in 1978.

The details of the project were complicated, but the overall concept was simple. If a referred patient was determined to be appropriate for Homemaker Service and/or Adult Day Care Health Services, the patient was randomly placed into either a test group, referred to as the expanded Medicare benefits group, or into a control group. The expanded benefits group patient was then referred for Homemaker Service and/or Adult Day Care Health Services, and these services were reimbursed on a pilot project basis by the Social Security Administration as additional Medicare benefits. If the patient was randomly selected into the control group, the referral source was notified that the patient did not qualify for these *additional* Medicare benefits, but did retain his eligibility for all presently existing Medicare benefits. In the case of a control patient, the referral source then set up a plan of care for the control group patient based upon the presently available and funded resources.

The fundamental aim of the project was to determine how the expanded 222 program, which included preventive as well as curative components of health care, compared to the control group type of case, which was the traditional curative care only.

After the project had been completed, the following report was issued:

Weissert, William, Thomas Wan, and Barbara Livieratos:
EFFECTS AND COSTS OF DAY CARE AND HOMEMAKER
SERVICES FOR THE CHRONICALLY ILL: A RANDOMIZED
EXPERIMENT.
National Center for Health Services Research, Dept. of Health,
Education and Welfare, DHEW Publication (PHS) 79-3250,
August, 1979.

In essence, the report questioned the cost effectiveness of the two alternatives to the traditional Medicare treatment. To state it differently, the report stated that the project did not demonstrate that prevention (homemaker services and day health care) was any more effective than cure. Not everyone agreed with these findings, however. For example, the following entities expressed grave doubts as to the validity of the government's conclusions:

Dept. of Health Services, State of California
    Fordham University, School of Social Work
    Office of Policy Analysis, Health Care Financing
    Administration (federal)

San Francisco Home Health Service
(largest of the six sites participating in the experimental
program)
On Lok Senior Health Service, San Francisco
Adult Day Health Services, State of Massachusetts
Maryland Department of Health and Mental Hygiene

When the smoke cleared away, the federal government was able to assume a virtuous attitude one more time. "Well, the Senate says Medicare is too restrictive. We instituted a program to test the consequences of removing some of the restrictions. It didn't work. Our report says so. Disregard the critics of our report." And so, to no one's surprise, the restrictions are still in place.

As mentioned earlier, at first the federal government reimbursed the home health agency, either nonprofit or profit making, after the service had been provided. The reimbursement rate was established on the basis of regulations defining "reasonable cost," which invariably turned out to be less than actual cost, unless of course fraud was involved. This resulted in the necessity for a nonprofit agency to resort to a fund-raising program. And, as I shall describe in a subsequent chapter, it sometimes led to fraud. Later the reimbursement, as in the case of hospitals, became prospective, subject to audit.

Administrative Deficiencies

Medicaid, the state equivalent of Medicare, partly financed by the federal government, reimburses agencies at less than "reasonable cost." In California, the rate of reimbursement is set forth in what is called a "schedule of maximum allowances," prepared in a mysterious way from mysterious sources.

In San Francisco, when agencies bid to obtain a contract to provide home health services to residents of the County of San Francisco under Title XX of the Social Security Act (Medicare is under Title XVII and Medicaid under Title XIX), the State of California, with a stupidity characteristic of many governmental bodies, insists that the contracts go to the lowest hourly bidders. This sounds reasonable until one understands what that means. For example, if one agency delivers 20 hours of service to a patient at an hourly rate of $10, when only 10 hours of service are needed, the agency that delivers only 10 hours of service at an hourly rate of $15 is saving the county $50 per month. One of my clients, an agency that demonstrated that its history of service to county residents resulted in lower costs to the county, nevertheless did not get a contract renewal because its *hourly* rate was higher than that of competitors, whose services cost more per month. When cost reports by home health agencies are audited by governmental personnel or certified public accounting firms, the results frequently leave much to be desired. I have personally been involved in cases in which the auditing personnel were ignorant of the Medicare laws and regulations, neglected to audit visit statistics, misplaced decimal points (25 hours of service being listed as 2.5 hours in the computer printout). Never have I seen an auditor who observed a home health care visit, or even thought it desirable to do so.

But perhaps the worst aspect of the situation is that the program has been so poorly publicized that most people are not even aware than it exists. The results are horrendous indeed. Here are some of them:

* People who could live relatively happily at home are sent to hospitals and nursing homes that are vastly more expensive.
* In the institutions that are often no better than filthy warehouses, they wither away and die.
* The relatives, who have their own lives to lead, are burdened with duties they have neither time nor knowledge to perform.
* The cost of institutional care is so prohibitively expensive that patients and their relatives find it difficult, if not impossible, to cope with the problem.
* In some areas, there are virtually no beds for those who need them.
* While government officials, news media, and the populace in general rant about the high cost of medical care, no real attempt is made to expand home health care, which has the potential of saving billions of dollars.

And who is at fault here? Most governmental agencies, physicians, hospitals and nursing homes seeking patients, the news media, and our elected officials. The American Institute of Certified Public Accountants and the equivalent state societies run seminars for accountants, teaching them how to maximize reimbursement, a euphemism for raising medical costs, while at the same time paying lip service to cost containment. And the overall problem is still— *waste.*

Hospice Services

The hospice program as presently practiced in the United States is relatively new. In one sense this seems surprising because the concept of hospice goes back a number of centuries. The term is one of a series of related words such as hospice, hostel, hotel, host, hospital, hospitaler, etc., all concerned with the very old practice of caring for the traveler, the sick, the aged, or to generalize it, the person in need of health care and shelter. The program dates back to medieval times, when the hospice (and the hospitalers) provided a resting place for crusaders returning from their travels.

As used originally in the United States, it was a program for terminally ill patients, usually suffering from cancer. These patients had a life expectancy of six months or less. With the development of the AIDS epidemic, a new and alarming caseload was thrust upon the hospices, which were totally unprepared financially and medically to deal with it. That emergency will be discussed in a subsequent chapter.

The Right to Die with Dignity

For cancer patients, the emphasis of hospice service was not to prolong life at any cost by medical treatment but to help the patient die with dignity and the diminution of pain and anxiety to the maximum extent possible.

The first and most famous modern hospice, St. Christopher's, was founded in London in 1967, by Dr. Cicely Saunders, with the assurance of two-thirds of its annual budget to be provided by the National Health Service.[4] Its excellent program involving the family of the dying patient, nursing care on a one-to-one basis, ready accessibility, bereavement services, etc., has been a model for modern hospices in other countries, including the United States. In 1974 Hospice, Inc., the first American hospice, situated in Connecticut, accepted its first patient. As of 1985, the number of American hospice care programs reached a total of over 1800.[5]

My involvement in the hospice program began in the 1970s, when one of the first hospice organizations was established in San Francisco. Shortly after inception, it was merged with the San Francisco Home Health Service, which had been a client of mine for a number of years. When I term the relationship a merger, I must explain that although each organization (both nonprofit) had its own board of directors, they shared office space and some personnel.

Hospices do not all follow the same pattern. Some provide in-patient care only, others concentrate on care for patients in their homes and offer a few hospital beds as backup, and still others combine the two methods.

However organized, they share many characteristics. They utilize an interdisciplinary team, consisting of an administrator, physician, nurse, social worker, homemaker/home health aides, therapists and other consultants and volunteers.[6] They provide service seven days a week, 24 hours a day. In addition, they offer consultation to the patient's family, preparing it to deal with the dying relative, and providing bereavement services after the patient's death.

The traditional medical method of treating a patient in pain is to allow the pain to develop until it has worsened to the point that the sufferer asks for the nurse who administers the appropriate drug at his or her earliest convenience. The hospice approach is to administer carefully measured dosages before the pain begins. In this way it is possible to avoid the memory and fear of pain, thus enabling the patient to review his or her life in peace, and come to terms with approaching death. The concept of preventing addiction to drugs should be considered meaningless when the patient has only a short time to live.

In England the emphasis has been to treat patients mainly in institutions, whereas in the United States, home care is the norm. In both countries the presence of relatives and friends is encouraged.

One reason the program has become important at this time is that our society to a large extent has moved away from the extended family to the nuclear family. Whereas formerly a dying parent or grandparent was cared for by the younger members of his or her family, today that is seldom the case, although it may still be practiced by some minority ethnic groups in the United States. Even in those cases, however, the emotional support may be undermined by the depressed economic status of the minority groups.

The Government Discovers That Dying Can Be Serious

Until October 1983, the government practically ignored the hospice movement. It took the position that the terminally ill patient was no different from other ill people. Medicare coverage from the point of view of allowable visits and reimbursement rates was the same for both. However, a new provider could be granted an exception (higher rates) for the first three years of its existence if such a higher rate could be substantiated. It is obvious that the costs would be, and in fact were, higher for hospice patients because of the weakness of the patients and the greater medical attention required.

The fiscal intermediaries, whether Blue Cross, Aetna, or some other insurance company, are by regulation supposed to assist the providers. In practice, however, the relationship becomes an adversarial one, with the fiscal intermediary demanding all kinds of special reports that frequently are not well explained and in most cases not understood by the providers. Never does the insurance company, which is supposed to help, actually visit the provider with an offer to assist.

They threaten, withhold or stop reimbursement, and in general discourage the provider—and in some cases force the provider out of business.

Until November 1, 1983, hospice services were considered to be part of the normal Medicare home health agency coverage, although certain special allowances were taken into account. On November 1, 1983, a new benefit specifically expanded the scope of Medicare to include the hospice benefit as the result of the passage of Section 122 of the Tax Equity and Fiscal Responsibility Act (TEFRA) of 1982. The final rules were published in the Federal Register December 16, 1983, by the Department of Health and Human Services (HHS). The rules defined services and set rates, subject to local area wage-level adjustments for routine home care, continuous home care, inpatient respite care (to relieve tired relatives temporarily) and inpatient care (usually terminal).

If any service is not reimbursed to the provider because the fiscal intermediary, such as Blue Cross, determines that the service rendered in good faith for some reason is not considered to be allowable, the cost will be borne by the provider, causing serious cash flow problems and, in extreme cases, bankruptcy. One of the reasons some expenditures were disallowed by governmental and fiscal intermediary personnel was that they seemed to think TEFRA, 1982, created terminal cancer. They could not be convinced that long before the hospice program was established, home health agency patients dying of cancer were being treated and the expenditures were being allowed. It is obvious that professional nursing service for the dying, whether the patient is being treated by a hospice or a home health agency, is more costly because the patient is weak and terminally ill.

Homemaker/Home Health Aide Service in the United States, written by Brahna Trager, defines the need for professional services as follows:

The Need for Professional Services

Those who are physically ill may have direct care needs, prescribed initially by the physician; sometimes with additions suggested by the staff as a result of assessment. Professional services, such as those for provision of medication, dressing changes, and other nursing procedures are scheduled as a part of the nursing plan. It may appear that the physical arrangement of the household is such that ambulation could be improved by use of a walker; or that physical therapy would increase the possibility that household equipment could be managed.

Direct services from professional health care personnel have their counterpart in the psychosocial status of the family or individual. *There may be profound post-hospital depression, or apprehension due to the sense of inadequacy so frequently associated with major physical changes. These problems often require regular supportive interviews.* Bizarre behavior in children or adults may indicate the need for psychological evaluation and support. Other professional services (nutrition, counseling, speech, physical or occupational therapy) may be scheduled as a part of service plans. [Author's emphasis.][7]

It is clear that the counseling we are discussing has been considered a covered service, unless one maintains that dying is not a major physical change. HCFA is undoubtedly in error if it maintains that counseling for the dying was invented on November 1, 1983, and at that point became an uncovered service, not reimbursable.

To sum it up we may say that the reimbursement procedure is based upon what the *reimbursement manual* says. The enforcing personnel are guided by the manual and not by the intent or constitutionality of the law. This is exactly what I was told by a representative of HCFA during a conference when I was representing a hospice organization.

Such being the case, my advice to my readers is clear. If you intend to die in the near future, don't expect counseling. Die quietly, in a dignified fashion, expeditiously.

The matter of bereavement counseling service provided to the individual's family after the demise of the individual is an interesting subject. The federal regulations state that it is a required service but that the cost of it is not reimbursable.[8]

This programmatic non sequitur is another example of our

myopic approach to health care. To surviving relatives, the death of a loved one can be, and frequently is, the cause of severe depression and consequent illness requiring eventual expensive treatment paid for by Medicare or Medicaid. However, the cost of the bereavement program, which is designed to prevent such depression and illness at a relatively minimal cost, is not reimbursable by Medicare or Medicaid. Once again the dictum is "get sick first, then we'll help you. If you're still alive!"

The denial of reimbursement for a required service poses a very interesting question. If it is a *required* hospice service, why is it not reimbursable? This is not only illogical but, I believe, discriminatory and unconstitutional. Let me explain that.

Let us assume that my neighbor has terminal cancer and that I am a skilled nurse. No governmental agency, not even HCFA, can demand that I render skilled nursing, including counseling to that neighbor, if I am not reimbursed for it. And if I choose to render such service, no governmental agency, including HCFA, can *require* that I render bereavement counseling without reimbursement. I assume that there is no question about the correctness of both of these statements.

Now let us assume that I am the proprietor of a Medicare-approved home health agency providing hospice to only terminally ill patients. Let us assume that I, as a skilled nurse, provide hospice service, including counseling but not bereavement services to my neighbor. Can I then be required legally to render bereavement counseling free?

If so, why and how can this be defended legally? As an individual I have freedom of choice to do that. As an individual I have freedom of choice to perform a charitable act. Am I to understand that as the proprietor of an agency, I must lose that freedom? Is anyone else in the country *required* to perform unreimbursed charity? Is the Bill of Rights to be suspended in the case of a hospice organization? That is unconstitutional.

I do not wish to be misunderstood. I believe that bereavement counseling should be *required. And reimbursed.* Any other course will harm the terminally ill patient's surviving relatives, and may even deprive the terminally ill patient of the hospice services he or she needs if the hospice organization cannot finance the bereavement counseling.

To phrase it differently, by requiring unreimbursed bereavement counseling, the program as written is unconstitutional and may very well destroy the whole intent of Congress.

It is essential before leaving the subject that we explore the role of governmental agencies in matters that relate to hospice but also go far beyond it. As mentioned earlier, most hospice patients are suffering from cancer, which is a group of over 100 related diseases that may arise in any of the body's tissues and that are characterized by the uncontrolled and disorderly multiplication of abnormal cells. In the United States, cancer is the second leading cause of death.[9]

Although much is unknown about the genesis and malignant development of cancer, some things we do know. A number of chemicals, radiation, genetic factors, repeated trauma, viruses to some extent, all of these separately or in a variety of combinations can be carcinogenic. It is the clear responsibility of governments to make every effort to eliminate the causative agents wherever possible. But what have the federal and state agencies done about it? Very little. This aspect of the problem will be examined in some detail later in the book.

The administration of the hospice program by the United States government is so severely flawed by restrictive and illogical legal requirements that the United States General Accounting Office (GAO) studied the problems and issued a report to the Subcommittee on Health, Committee on Ways and Means, House of Representatives, in September 1989.[10] The purpose of the study was to determine why only about 35% of the estimated 1700 hospice organizations participate in Medicare. In brief the GAO reported that one-half of the nonparticipating hospices sampled said their main concerns were:

- The physicians required to report on patients had to certify that a patient is terminally ill and will die within six months. Hospice officials state that physicians favor modification of the certification language to state that the patient is terminally ill and will die within six months "if the terminal disease runs its normal course." The reason for this proposed change is to allow for the obvious uncertainties involved in long-term prognosis.
- It is required that hospice organizations obtain contracts with hospitals for inpatient services. In some cases this is impracticable, particularly in rural areas.
- The limit placed on aggregate payments for individual patients ($9,010) was not always reasonable where the six-month maximum period was exceeded.
- 76% of the hospice officials queried think that the exclusion of

Medicare payment for bereavement counseling after the patient's death adversely affects hospice operations.
- Participating hospices felt that a two-day limit to obtain a physician's terminal-illness certification after the day of the patient's admission to a hospice should be extended to eight days.

The Hospice Association of America responded to the GAO report on August 7, 1989. In general the response agreed with the recommendations of GAO, but it included a few additional recommendations. One was that home care nurses (also trained in hospice care) could move into a hospice program, eliminating the need for a separate nursing staff. Another comment was that the reimbursement rates were inadequate because they had been set in 1986, and costs were higher in 1989.

Of all these recommendations, the only one that was put into effect was the extension of the two-day physician certifications from two days to eight days.

As Horace wrote in *Ars Poetica,* "The mountains will be in labor, and a ridiculous mouse will be brought forth."

Considering the number of terminally ill people in the United States, there is no doubt that the hospice program should be a very important component of a national health care system, but what conclusions can we draw as to its fiscal management?

The tragic truth is that an enormous proportion of funds expended on hospice care arises from the fact that our government itself is responsible for much of the cancer resulting from avoidable smoking, industrial pollution, and substandard living conditions of large segments of the population.

Of the estimated 1,700 hospices in the country (GAO's estimate), we have noted that only 35% participate in the Medicare program because of restrictive requirements that abort the effectiveness of the expenditures made and may even force hospice organizations into bankruptcy. In either case the result is that terminally ill patients are compelled to seek help in acute care facilities or in nursing homes, both of which are far more expensive and not geared to render proper hospice care.

5. AIDS

In June, 1981, a friend visited my wife and me in our home in California. He was a very intelligent, cultured psychiatrist who had been living and practicing in the Midwest and was in the process of moving to southern California. Generally he made no attempt to deny his homosexuality, although his family was apparently not aware of it. He was suffering from symptoms that his doctors and he himself did not understand. His chronic exhaustion and general developing debilitation led him to believe that he had systemic lupus erythematosus, normally called lupus, about which very little is known, but it is clear that it is what is termed an autoimmune disease, which means that in a way, the individual becomes allergic to parts of his/her own body. The afflicted people have a myriad of symptoms that come and go with frustrating unpredictability, causing severe suffering and disorientation, and making diagnosis extremely difficult. We thought he was probably a hypochondriac.

He settled in Los Angeles, and as time progressed he developed chronic diarrhea and a number of skin rashes, but managed to continue practicing his profession. By September of 1984, however, his condition dramatically deteriorated, and he contracted idiopathic thrombocytopenic purpura (ITP), which can be defined as a low number of platelets involved in normal blood clotting. He died in December 1984, while his lungs were being examined by bronchoscopy. I believe he was among the first identified casualties of AIDS in the United States, and although I have known subsequent casualties of the dread disease, I have never recovered from the shock of that first one.

What Is AIDS?

To most of the country, until Rock Hudson died of AIDS on October 2, 1985, AIDS was considered a faceless malady afflicting anonymous male homosexuals (gays), but if a famous actor who was a friend of President Reagan and the idol of millions of women (and men too) could die of it, it must be serious indeed. This disorder, acquired immune deficiency syndrome, kills its victims by destroying or severely damaging their immune systems, particularly the T-helper cells that normally fight infections, and thus shield people against disease. The problem here is that the retrovirus that causes AIDS is at this period rampant and there is no known vaccine to prevent its deadly attack, complicated by the fact that like other viruses, but perhaps to a greater degree, it has the ability to mutate, which severely hampers the ability of the immune system to combat it.

The afflicted individuals die of a variety of infections, which would not have developed if the T-helper cells were operating properly. One of the important diseases is Kaposi's sarcoma (KS), which was a form of cancer discovered originally among Italian and Jewish men from the Mediterranean area in 1871, striking them in their 40s and 50s.[1] According to reports documented in medical books of the 19th century, it was fairly benign; not so in AIDS patients. KS is frequently the forerunner of other opportunistic infections, which are the killers, one of the most common of which is pneumocystis carinii pneumonia. Other killers are microorganisms that do not ordinarily cause disease.

AIDS-related complex (ARC) has been since 1985 the term used to describe infected patients who have many other symptoms, including weight loss, fevers, fatigue, night sweats, diarrhea, swollen glands, and T-cell disorders. It is not full-fledged AIDS but may later develop into it. As this is not a medical text, I shall proceed no further with a discussion of technicalities or tests associated with it, other than to say that the current definition of AIDS per the Center for Disease Control (CDC) is that anyone with a T-helper count of 200 or less and/or the presence of AIDS-defining opportunistic infection or malignancy, regardless of helper count, has AIDS.

The Scope of the Problem

AIDS was first discovered in Africa in the 1970s, but because of the inadequate reports emanating from that continent it is impossible to estimate the number of cases there at this time. In the United States since 1981, when it was first identified, the number of cases has increased dramatically; by February 1989 the reported cases amounted to 86,000 in the mainland United States and an additional 2,000 in our possessions.[2] In 1989, 40,000 Americans had died of the disease. By 1991, well over 100,000 Americans had died of AIDS and an estimated one million are currently infected with the virus, of whom 125,000 are thought to have clinical AIDS. In many other countries there is a stubborn denial that homosexuality exists, and consequently they report few, if any, cases of AIDS. The most frightening aspect of the epidemic is discussed by Stephen Jay Gould, a professor of biology at Harvard University.[3] In his opinion it has probably reached a saturation point in Africa, but is increasing exponentially in the rest of the world. Stated simply, that means that in a population of billions, when 1 case increases to 2, or 2 to 4, that merits little attention. But when 1 million increases to 2 million, and 2 million to 4 million, that is a different and horrifying prospect.

A report called "AIDS in the World" was prepared by a Harvard-based international group of experts called the Global AIDS Policy Coalition, headed by Dr. Jonathan Mann, director of Harvard's International AIDS Center. As reported in the *San Francisco Chronicle* June 4, 1992, it states that:

1. In less than three more years, the worldwide total of infected adults is bound to rise from nearly 12 million today to 17.5 million in 1995.
2. Women constitute the fastest-growing group of HIV-infected people worldwide, rising from 25% of all HIV cases two years ago to 40% today.
3. The unchecked virus will strike no fewer than 38 million adults, and quite possibly as many as 110 million, before the end of the decade (not including at least 10 million children who will also become infected within the next few years).

Some Sociological Influences

As mentioned, AIDS in this country has been primarily an epidemic of gays, but women who have sexual relations with infected men, whether the women are prostitutes or not, children born of infected mothers, and individuals who receive infected blood transfusions may also contract the disease. Currently, the most rapid growth of new infections is to be found among black and Hispanic IV drug users sharing dirty needles. Incidentally, it is estimated that in parts of Africa 40% of the heterosexual population is infected with AIDS.[4] In some areas of central Africa, 10% to 20% of the general population and up to 80% of the prostitutes are infected with AIDS, and it is estimated that half the cases in Africa are found in heterosexual women.[5]

Homosexuality has been recorded as an ancient and universal form of sexual behavior.[6] In ancient Greece it was accepted and in some cases encouraged. Some of history's more famous examples include Alexander the Great, Leonardo Da Vinci, Michelangelo Buonarroti, Walt Whitman, James Baldwin, Sappho of Lesbos, Oscar Wilde, Allen Ginsberg, Herman Melville, and Thomas Mann. The world would have been a sorry place without them.

Nevertheless, it is a matter of common knowledge that to a large segment of the American public, homosexuality is immoral and condemned by the Judeo-Christian ethic. As a result, AIDS is considered the just punishnent of the sinners. Unfortunately this attitude in some cases impinges on the victims themselves. According to the *San Francisco Chronicle,* March 7, 1991, violence against gays and lesbians rose sharply in 1990, aggregating 425 attacks and other acts of harassment, increasing 28% from 1989. Nationally the increase in major cities amounted to 42%. However, it is undoubtedly an over-simplification to attribute this hostility to morals alone; a few such acts spring from a desire to deny the homosexual tendencies of the perpetrators of those acts. Homophobia is not a simple act. In addition many such acts, as in the case of rape, are never reported.

There is no known cure for AIDS at present, but there are drugs such as AZT and ddI that can clearly prolong life and may prevent certain of the opportunistic infections. However, fear affects many associated with it, or potentially associated with it, whether patients, lovers, family members, friends, gays who are apparently not infected, some doctors, dentists, other medical personnel or people wishing to help those infected. In some cases, in spite of their ethical standards, physicians who traditionally have put the patients' interests first have refused to treat some of the patients. Although there is no reliable information as to the number of physicians and nurses who refuse to treat such patients, some of them do not demonstrate the courage and dedication necessary.[7] It should be stressed that they are the exceptions rather than the rule.

Another problem was the lack of early treatment of the disease; one of the reasons for this was lack of knowledge about how to treat it, but there was more to it than that. There was clear evidence of discrimination. For example, the NIH's spending for Legionnaire's disease in the early 1980s cost $34,841 for each legionnaire's death, contrasting with $3,225 per AIDS death, indicating clearly that to the government the life of a gay man was worth a small fraction of the life of a member of the American Legion![8]

Outreach was poorly organized. In 1987, C. Everett Koop, U.S. Surgeon General, made some excellent suggestions such as AIDS education in the schools and condom advertisements on television, and he asked President Reagan to take a leading role in fighting the epidemic.[9] Most of this came to nought. Reagan was unmoved. Material issued to the public in pamphlets was couched in polite language not understood by the readers; many of the readers could not read the language used, and many were illiterate. Outreach needed a more person-to-person, down-to-earth approach. And of course there were the moral objections to bringing up the condom issue. That would encourage sex. What about movies, television, sexy advertisements of women and men wearing scanty underwear, touting perfumes and deodorants? Is that intended to promote celibacy? Another example of this type of shortsightedness was and is the refusal to issue clean needles to IV drug users to prevent the spread of the epidemic through the sharing of infected needles. There is no way to sum up all this nonsense other than to say that the money spent to fight the epidemic was not only inadequate but wasted because of lack of a sensible approach to the problem.

Because it is regarded as a gay disease, most heterosexuals feel that gays should fight it. The homosexual community rose to the challenge magnificently; they established nonprofit organizations to raise money, lobby for governmental assistance, educate the public, provide care for the afflicted AIDS and HIV-positive people, and in general do whatever they could to help. In effect they tried to accomplish what the national and local governments should have been doing. Unfortunately, the cost was excessive. Some of the executives did not have the skills and education necessary to run complicated programs and organizations, and the stresses were so grievous that rapid burnout and turnover were inevitable. But it should be stressed that there are many areas of success, such as the dramatic decrease of newly acquired HIV infections in some groups in the gay community, the establishment of patient and health care community centers, etc.

Where the Big Bucks Are

One of the more sinister aspects of the AIDS epidemic is the fact that big money and big prestige are available to the actors in the drama. This is particularly applicable to physicians, researchers, pharmaceutical companies and insurance companies. Government bureaucrats frequently lack the principles or desire to curb abuses. The scenario is not much different from the Iran-Contra scandal or the savings and loan disaster.

In the world of science, certain diseases can make careers, and AIDS is one of those. For the smart operators, Nobel Prizes, reputations and remunerative lifetime careers can be the rewards. Dr. Robert Gallo, the chief of the Laboratory of Tumor Cell Biology at the National Cancer Institute, was reported by the U.S. government to have discovered and isolated the AIDS virus at the end of 1983.[10] However, in April of 1983, Dr. Luc Montagnier at the Pasteur Institute in Paris claimed that *he* had discovered the virus. He called it lymphadenopathy-associated virus (LAV).[11] In the spring of 1990 the NIH became interested and instituted an investigation.[12] The question was whether Dr. Gallo had erroneously claimed as his own discovery the virus he had received from Paris.

Nobel Prize-winning biologist David Baltimore participated in research and coauthored a report on the body's immune system.[13] In March 1991, he asked that the paper be withdrawn from publication in a scientific journal because he had been accused of making assertions as to the veracity of experiments he had accepted without evidence to support them.

Burroughs Wellcome, the global pharmaceutical company, sells over two billion dollars of drug products annually. It also has a U.S. subsidiary which, by 1986, had been developing AZT at a cost of over $50 million. AZT is the only approved drug to materially help AIDS patients, but the original cost of $10,000 per year per patient was the highest price in history for a drug.[14] The cost has been reduced to a "mere" $3,000–$5,000, and will be paid by most insurance companies, *if the patient has coverage*, and many do not. Medicaid does not cover cost, and demands that the patient's funds be spent down before coverage begins. For many, many AIDS patients, the world is not just grim—it is terrifying.

Disastrous events are not the exception in our world; they occur regularly—earthquakes, wars, floods, tornadoes, hurricanes, fires, tidal waves, etc. Some we may be able to predict, some we cannot, some (few) can be prevented, most cannot. If we prepare properly, we can reduce the damage to life and property. That, however, takes very careful planning, knowledge, and discipline. Architectural improvements, erecting barriers where appropriate, providing in advance for supplies, food, medicines, and medical care by trained experts are needed to enable a community to survive after the event and until normalcy returns. Escape routes in many cases and other contingencies must be taken care of during and after the crises. An excellent example of how to approach the problem can be found in an article in *The New England Journal of Medicine,* Vol. 324, No. 12, March 21, 1991. It is entitled "Disaster Planning and Response," by Joseph F. Waekerle, M.D.

In the case of the AIDS epidemic, it is true, of course, that planning for such an unusual, unpredictable disease was not possible in advance. However, an efficient health system should be able to mobilize its forces to cope with such an emergency, if it has as its goal the welfare of people, and not the protection of the medical establishment, the pharmaceutical companies, etc. If it blunders around myopically, the money spent is, to a large extent, wasted.

Ten years into the AIDS epidemic the price in human suffering and death and the financial costs have already been enormous. Key cities such as New York and San Francisco have felt the heaviest impact and have had to be subsidized, even if inadequately, by federal and state agencies. But the costs continue to increase and are now becoming evident in smaller and less organized cities throughout the country. In addition, as noted before, the epidemic is rapidly spreading into the black and Hispanic communities. Historically, these groups have been woefully underserved by our health care system and are now becoming an increasing drain on our health and fiscal resources, and may well push our already tottering system over the edge.

There are clearly two main concerns that must be addressed over and beyond the immediate and overwhelming medical care and other needs of AIDS and ARC patients. The first of these is research into the cure and prevention of the disease itself. This issue has already been addressed by some of the most sophisticated laboratories, but the people working on it need concentrated and massive financial backing similar to or even greater than our support of space exploration and colonization. The scientific establishment needs to be freed from the daily struggle to corral grants, find adequate staff, and obtain needed supplies. It must be turned loose to go all out and in the course of its efforts it will not only find the cure to AIDS, but will add mightily to the knowledge about cancer and many other diseases.

The second prong of the attack must be prevention. Petty and unproven moralistic arguments about sex instruction for the schoolchild, about clean needle exchange encouraging drug use, and condom use encouraging sex must be discarded. An all-out campaign that will reach out to the uneducated, the ignorant and the illiterate must be mounted. At present, pending a cure, which may be a long way off, this is the only means to prevent untold suffering and save billions of dollars that will otherwise be spent on fruitless care.

The inadequacy of our nation's effort to deal with the crisis cannot be overemphasized. Here are a few of the shortcomings:

1. AIDS has been a low government priority from 1982 to 1984, with the following Public Health Service funding:

1982	$5.4 million
1983	28.06 million
1984	61.4 million

   This was a pitiful attempt to deal with a problem that was to cost tens of thousands of lives.[15]
2. All of the major clinical trials have excluded women, minorities, and IV drug users. What we know clinically is based on studies of white homosexual males.
3. Ten years into the epidemic, AZT remains the *only* approved drug for treatment. With more research funds we might have been further along.
4. Ulcerating sexually transmitted diseases like syphilis, chancroid, and herpes dramatically increase the likelihood of transmission of HIV, yet funding to clinics treating these diseases has decreased, in spite of the rapid increases in these sexually transmitted diseases during the 1980s.

Not even Franz Kafka, with his genius for describing in harrowing detail the frustrations of trying to deal with a malignant bureaucracy, as he did in *The Castle* or *The Trial*, could have devised a worse scenario. The only conclusion we can draw is that the money spent on AIDS up to now has to a large extent been wasted because it has been too little, too late, and too unfocused.

6. Alternative Health Care Financing

National health insurance has as its goal health care services for all the people in the United States. As we have seen in the preceding chapters, the private acute care hospitals, whether nonprofit or proprietary, the county hospitals, the nursing homes, the in-home services, all had crucial deficiencies when judged by their ability to deliver adequate health care services to our total population. Before launching into this disquisition on health care alternatives, allow me to define the overall key problem. The American Medical Association, the American Hospital Association, the governmental agencies, the pharmaceutical companies, in fact all health providers, agencies, and their advisers have refused to consider national health insurance as a viable solution. They try to erect an edifice without a foundation. They continue to devise, as Gilbert and Sullivan put it, in desperation, "a thing of shreds and patches." In this chapter we shall analyze three of those—Medicare and Medicaid, veterans' hospitals, and health maintenance organizations.

Medicare and Medicaid

Attitudes toward health policies in the United States during the early 1930s changed rapidly and drastically as the AMA, the AHA, politicians, and various segments of the general populace attempted to deal with the ravages of the Great Depression. Movements toward some form of national health insurance were embraced and eschewed with bewildering rapidity.[1] Eventually, a federal program of grants-in-aid to the states for old age assistance (OAA) was instituted by the passage of Title I of the Social Security Act of 1935. It was extremely important because it prohibited the use of those grants to finance care for inmates of a public institution. In other words, it established the practice of assistance to people by cash grants rather than by supporting institutions to house them. A national health conference was held in 1938,[2] which brought together a wide spectrum of people interested in public health; it was the first truly national discussion

of the subject. In 1939, Democratic senator Robert F. Wagner drafted
a bill outlining a far-reaching federal health program, providing for
federal grants-in-aid to states for state medical care programs
designed by each state. It was widely discussed but never brought to
a vote. Other bills, such as the Wagner-Murray-Dingell Bill, the
Green-Eliot Bill, and the Taft Bill were drafted, differing in some
ways from each other but all attempting to provide a comprehensive
approach to the subject of public health. They were discussed extensively but did not become law.

As discussed in Chapter 1, the Hill-Burton Act was passed in
1946, and although it was not enforced until 1972 and even then in an
inadequate manner, its philosophical impact was positive in that it
brought forth the idea that the indigent had a *right* to medical care,
even if insufficient.

In 1960 Congress established the Kerr-Mills program, which
extended federal support for welfare medical programs in the United
States (a federal matching program). It was a step forward, but did
not reach the great majority of needy people.

Medicare and Medicaid—The Good—The Bad

The real far-reaching change came in 1965 when Congress
enacted two new programs—Medicare and Medicaid (Titles XVIII
and XIX respectively of the Social Security Act). Medicare provided
the population 65 years and older with hospital and other medical
benefits. Basically these at first included up to 90 days of hospital
care, post-hospital care in a skilled nursing home, home health services, and physician services. There were some deductibles, and payment to providers was on the basis of "reasonable costs." Medicaid
was a state program by which states were mandated to set up
programs to provide comprehensive care for those unable to pay, with
the federal government providing matching funds to the states based
upon the financial status of each state. The program also included
other welfare recipients such as Aid to the Blind, Aid to Disabled, and
Aid to Families with Dependent Children.

It is difficult to assess the importance of Medicare and Medicaid.
For the first time, we saw medical care for the elderly and the poor as
a *right* and not a charitable gift to the "deserving" poor. To politicians
and the AMA, the word "right" is synonymous with "anathema,"
particularly when in the hands of the poor. The doctor has the right
to charge what the traffic will bear, the right to admit or not admit a

patient to a hospital, and the exclusive right to prescribe medicines. The government servant has the right to flout the law and become a national hero and a highly paid public speaker like Oliver North. One way to defuse the dangerous word "right" is to refer to it as a slightly unclean "entitlement."

At the inception of Medicaid, the states were mandated to provide comprehensive medical care for everyone unable to pay. Each state was to decide how to run its program. The states could also decide to cover any of the acceptable welfare categories even if the individual's income or assets were too large to receive welfare, but not large enough for him/her to pay for care.

In theory, the coverage sounds completely comprehensive. In practice, however, many poor people were unable to receive coverage for medical services. Some of those were the following:

* People under 65 who were not blind, or parents of minor children; no matter how poor they were.
* Those whose income was low but still above the poverty levels. In the event of catastrophic illness, the only way for them to be covered was to spend their own money down to the poverty level. Then they could receive Medicaid funds.
* Most gas attendants, maids, and housekeepers working part-time.
* Seasonal workers.
* Migrant workers.
* Undocumented workers.

In addition to Medicare and Medicaid, there is also private health insurance coverage. However, taking all three types of coverage into account, a large number of people have no health insurance coverage of any kind. At the present time, it is estimated that about 37 million people are in that category.

One of the reasons for discussing the question of coverage here is to refute the claim by some health providers that Hill-Burton compliance was unimportant or even unnecessary because practically everyone in the United States has some form of health insurance. The indigent, who have no health insurance coverage, are still with us.

Another aspect of Medicaid that is mentioned here and will be touched upon later is that acute care hospitals have frequently claimed that Medicaid reimbursement for services rendered to Medicaid patients is so low that hospitals lose money, and then have to charge more for services rendered to other patients who pay their own bills or have better-paying insurance coverage.

This argument was put to the test in California at the beginning of 1983. In order to reduce Medi-Cal expenditures (California's name for Medicaid), California's Department of Health Services decided to select hospitals in several areas of California that should get Medi-Cal clients on a competitive bid basis. The hospitals suddenly discovered that when they lost Medi-Cal clients, they began to suffer a financial crisis. The reduction in volume of service left the hospitals with empty beds, which, as has been mentioned earlier, cost about two-thirds as much to maintain as occupied beds. To put it bluntly, Medicaid business is good for hospitals—all they want is higher reimbursement.

Contrary to popular belief, not all diseases are covered by Medicare and Medicaid. For example, a person suffering from Alzheimer's disease, a senile dementia sometimes occurring at an early age, is not eligible for financial aid under Medicare. At a congressional committee hearing in December 1983, Representative Claude Pepper, Democrat of Florida, chairman of the House Subcommittee on Health and Long-Term Care, stated:

> It's a terrible disease, the fourth largest killer in our society, and yet it's not covered by Medicare. A dreadful burden is placed on ordinary people when this horrible illness strikes.[3]

The problem, Pepper observed, is that Medicare is designed to take care of acute illnesses requiring hospitalization, while Alzheimer's is a long-term chronic ailment whose sufferers generally need care in their homes and sometimes in nursing homes. We are constantly being reminded that the American health care system is bankrupting the country, that poor people are being pampered by an overly liberal Medicare and Medicaid utilization. It *is* true that medical costs have risen at an alarming rate, higher indeed than the inflation rate characteristic of the rest of our economy. Let us look at some of the causes and make a few comparisons.

The *Wall Street Journal,* in discussing the 1984 Medicare scene, pointed out that Medicare finances hundreds of thousands of unnecessary operations but will not pay for inexpensive preventive measures, that proposals to increase deductibles and premiums will increase the burdens of hard-pressed taxpayers and elderly people, that the conversion of the Medicare system into a catastrophic coverage system would further aggravate the cost problem. The *Wall Street Journal* article concludes that we must forget the dreams and reform the entire system.[4]

And what of the claim that the poor people in the United States are being pampered? An article from the *Washington Post* states:

It is better to be poor in Sweden, France, West Germany, Australia, Israel, Canada, and Britain than in most of the United States, according to a Columbia University study.[5]

The three-year study was conducted by Alfred J. Kahn and Sheila B. Kamerman. In an interview amplifying the study, Kahn stated:

We are not doing very well by the families who are in financial difficulties, in contrast to most Western countries, including those who are much poorer.[6]

Other countries are much more generous in compensating for the high costs of rearing children: All eight countries studied except for the United States have child allowances. All except the United States and Australia have statutory maternity benefits. "Civilized societies everywhere except in the United States recognize that children are a valuable resource and we have a responsibility to make sure they grow up healthy," Kahn said. In Sweden, support payments to a single, unemployed mother with two children equal 93% of the income of the average worker in that country after taxes. The comparable figure for Pennsylvania, which is in the upper third of U.S. states in welfare benefits, is 44%. Ranking in generosity after Sweden and France (which provides 78.6% of its average worker's wage after taxes) are West Germany at 67.3%, Canada at 52.5%, Britain at 51.7% and Australia and Israel at 50%. Rebutting assertions that welfare mothers give birth in order to get aid, Kahn said, "The studies show there is no relationship between the generosity of a program and the birthrate. In every country, families without children are better off economically than families with children, and working families are better off than the unemployed. "

As for maternity benefits, this is the only country where the law does not require companies to replace working mothers' lost income to some degree. In 1978, Congress required employers who give disability insurance to allow mothers to collect maternity benefits under those programs. However, 60% of American working women still receive no income replacement during maternity leave. In Israel, by contrast, mothers receive 75% of their wages for 12 weeks through a combination of contributions from employer and government. Sweden provides 90% of lost income for nine months. West Germany provides benefits for 7 1/2 months, France for 16 weeks, Canada for 17 weeks, and Britain for 18 weeks.

It is indeed ironic that the United States, the richest country in the world, with a health care system riddled with inefficiency and corruption, unable to care for its poor people as well as other countries not nearly as rich, seeks a solution that will further impoverish the indigent and deny them needed health care services, while forcing the women to complete an unwanted or unplanned pregnancy.

Before leaving this subject it is important to understand the close interrelationships between physicians, hospitals, Medicare, Medicaid, governmental agencies, Blue Cross, Blue Shield, and several lesser health insurance companies. An excellent discussion can be found in *Blue Cross—What Went Wrong?* by Sylvia A. Law, Yale University Press, 1974. In the 1930s, hospitals, in serious financial trouble because of the Depression, were anxious to develop a stable method of being reimbursed for services. Blue Cross, created by hospitals and run by them, was the answer. The American Hospital Association, in close collaboration with the American Medical Association, was successful in securing enabling legislation to set standards for reimbursement of medical services. Blue Cross for payments to hospitals, and Blue Shield for payments to physicians, were firmly established as the regulating agencies. And when in 1965 Medicare and Medicaid were initiated, Blue Cross immediately became the fiscal intermediary (paying agency) for reimbursement.[7] Other health insurance companies also got a piece of the action, but to a minor extent. No complaints were heard that this was a clear conflict of interest, because the insurance companies, by making Medicare and Medicaid cumbersome and difficult, could make their own insurance in the health field look attractive by comparison and thus increase their policy sales.

From 1965 to 1984 the method of reimbursement was retrospective—that is, hospitals were reimbursed for "reasonable costs" determined after the fiscal year had ended, even though the term "reasonable costs" was a euphemism for whatever costs, reasonable or not, that the hospitals could get away with. The rapid increase of health care costs was phenomenal. For example, in 1965 health care accounted for 6% of G.N.P., increasing annually, reaching 10.5% in 1982 or $322 billion, of which approximately 27% was paid for by Medicare and Medicaid. The rate of inflation for health care costs in 1982 was 12.6%, three times the general rate of inflation.[8]

The runaway costs were countered by a new system of reimbursement—prospective payment. In brief, the new system established a preset rate per case or type of diagnosis. It characterizes discharges by a method known as diagnosis related group classification, or DRGs; 467 such categories were set up. This system was to be phased in beginning October 1, 1983, reaching completion in the fiscal year beginning October 1, 1986. Hospitals are paid the preset rate for each case of illness. If the hospital can provide the service at a lower rate it can pocket the saving. Two questions are appropriate at this time. One is, "Did the new prospective payment system curb inflation, or as the current phrase goes, did it effect 'cost containment'?" The answer is an unequivocal *no*. The consumer price index (CPI) is a measure of the average change in prices over time of basic consumer goods and services.[9] The following figures are prepared by the Bureau of Labor Statistics, U.S. Labor Department:

	Year		**% Increase by**
	1984	**1988**	**1988 over 1984**
Food and Beverages	103.2	118.2	14.54
Housing	103.6	118.5	14.39
Apparel and Upkeep	102.1	115.4	13.03
Transportation	103.7	108.7	4.83
Medical Care	106.8	138.6	29.78
Entertainment	103.8	120.3	15.90
Other Goods and Services*	107.9	137.0	26.97

*includes tobacco products, toilet goods, personal care

Obviously, cost containment of health care services is not working very well.

The second question is, "How well is the prospective payment working?" Not well, as will be explained in a subsequent chapter.

In 1988, Congress passed a measure granting those over 65 years of age certain special privileges if the annual income of a single person was no more than $6,620 or the income of a couple was no more than $8,880.[10] The privileges included an exemption from paying the $30 monthly insurance premium, the elimination of paying a $728 share of each hospital stay and the 20% of the doctor's fee for Medicare beneficiaries. However, the Social Security Administration and the Health Care Financing Administration failed to let more than 55% of the eligible people know that the benefits existed, and so the government continues to deduct the premiums from the Social Security checks, and the hospital's $728 and the doctor's 20% are still paid for by the elderly. Why? The government claims that it is difficult to know who is entitled to the benefits. When it is a question of collecting income taxes, the government does not have any difficulty in knowing who is liable for taxes. As Henry Waxman, Democrat of California and chairman of the House Committee on Health and the Environment, put it:

> Saying the poor, elderly people are out of luck if they don't know the program exists because the government isn't going to tell them is disgraceful.

Or as Senator Edward M. Kennedy, Democrat of Massachusetts and chairman of the Senate Labor and Human Resources Committee, said:

> The administration can clearly do more to notify senior citizens of their rights. Seniors should not be denied the medical care they need because the bureaucracy has failed to do its job.

If one contends that by not granting exemptions to the elderly, the government is illegally saving health care money, it is simply a question of the old shell game. The health care expenditure is incurred, but this time by the people who are supposed to be the recipients.

The Paper Labyrinth

Talk to any physician or other health care practitioner who is attempting to provide services to Medicaid patients and you will be subjected to a diatribe of gargantuan proportions. To get paid for operating on an ingrown toenail will consume filling out and submitting (usually resubmitting as well) paper forms that sometimes defy understanding. What frequently happens is that the practitioner will cease to treat Medicaid patients or will do so, if he/she is sufficiently dedicated, and the time is not prohibitive, without even asking to be paid. And if that happens often, he/she will charge more to the patients who can afford to pay.

The whole procedure can be a colossal waste of time, money, and talent.

Veterans' Hospitals

Veterans' hospitals constitute a much greater proportion of our country's medical system than most people realize. To place it in perspective, it should be noted that the Veterans Administration in 1988 had a net outlay of $29,244 billion.[11] It operates 170 hospitals, with nearly 100,000 beds and one million patients treated annually. Presumably the beneficiaries of this mammoth program are the American veterans; how have they fared?

The Revolutionary War

Since the birth of the United States the lot of the American war veteran has not been a happy one. Promises of the rewards to the veterans were not lacking—proposed salaries, land and cash bonuses after the Revolution were lavish but evanescent. Some of the veterans attempted to remedy the situation. The most famous of these was Daniel Shays, who was born in 1747 of poor Irish Protestant parents.[12] With little education he managed to purchase some farmland, but once the war started he enlisted, was wounded, decorated for valor and was eventually presented with an ornamental sword by the Marquis de Lafayette in recognition of his conspicuous bravery during battle.

After the war he returned to his farm, but was so short of cash that he was taken to court several times, once because he was unable to pay a debt of £12 and again for a debt of £3. In one respect he was lucky; other veterans ended up in debtors' prison.

In 1786–87, Shays led a group of about 1200 debt-ridden farmers in western Massachusetts to protest the adjournment of the legislature before action was taken to halt many farm foreclosures.[13] Several marches were repulsed by government troops, and Shays was termed the leader of "Shays's Rebellion."

The *Massachusetts Sentinel,* published in Boston, referred to protestors of this kind as follows: "Let us sweep them from the land—and since they do not know how to prize the blessing of equal law and liberty, let them be cut off, or exiled to those lands where no traitor can escape the punishment due his crimes."[14] The proposed punishment seems inappropriate because they had no blessings to prize and had already been exiled to debtors' prison.

The War of 1812 and the Mexican War

James Monroe, president of the United States from 1817 to 1825, himself wounded in the Revolutionary War, believed firmly that the country should provide for survivors of wars, particularly those who were reduced to indigence. This would comprise poor and infirm veterans, including those who had never been injured in the war. He also proposed a monthly pension plan for officers and enlisted men. There was a great deal of patriotic fervid expression but a minimum of action. Veterans were required to make a statement of indigence before they could qualify for pensions, and veterans on pensions could be stricken from the rolls if they had no proof of poverty.

The Civil War

The Civil War introduced a new and particularly ugly note into the already discordant cacophony of the veteran dirge. Before we get to that, however, let us look at the plight of the veterans in general. On August 5, 1865, the *New York Herald* published this letter from an unhappy veteran cavalryman:

What are the returned soldiers who volunteered to fight for their country and who were mustered out honorably from the service to do for employment? Are our wives and children to starve? All are willing to work, I am sure, if they can find employment. If a soldier asks for a situation, the response generally is, "We are full," or "We engaged a clerk this morning."[15]

And here is an advertisement in the same newspaper:

Wanted—by a young man who served in the army for three years, at anything he can make an honest living. Call 356 7th Avenue.

Many veterans in seeking employment chose not to mention the fact that they were veterans of the Civil War. The *Army and Navy Journal* advised veteran applicants in 1865 "not to slump and become a dirty loafer 'who has been in the army,' " and that if mutilated by war, "teach yourself the strategy of new muscular habits." In Chicago, Governor Richard Oglesby, at a reception to honor veterans, advised them to help themselves and not expect to be given "soup . . . with a silver spoon."

Black veterans, both in the North and in the South, were special targets of discrimination once the war was over. Just in time for Christmas, 1865, the Ku Klux Klan, deriving its name from "Koklos," the Greek word for "circle," was invented to "protect and defend the weak, the innocent, and defenseless," and "to protect and defend the Constitution of the United States." That was to be accomplished, presumably, by lynching blacks.

Such tiny bounties as were paid to veterans were far smaller for blacks than for whites.

During the Civil War, morphine, a derivative of opium, was injected into wounded soldiers by doctors with no alternatives; powdered opium with ipecac, laudanum, and paregoric (more than 2,800,000 ounces) were issued to the wounded, and when mustered from the service, the veterans became shunned and feared drug addicts.[16]

After the Civil War the military events in the United States were relatively minor until World War I, and in the aftermath of that war President Warren G. Harding transferred 57 hospitals then being operated by the U.S. Public Health Service to the Veterans Bureau, which eventually became the Veterans Administration.

The Unhappy Story of the Veterans' Hospitals

Within two years after its establishment, the Veterans Administration (VA) became involved in a scandal of epic proportions.[17] Funds were flagrantly misused and involved the private sale of medical supplies and extravagant land deals, ending in the suicide of the general counsel of the bureau and the conviction and imprisonment of its director, Colonel Charles Forbes. For a time, the VA lived in the land of oblivion, and attracted very few competent physicians. At the end of World War II, it came to life again, with the help of additional funds, doctors who had been in military service, and affiliations with medical schools. Unfortunately, to this day it has not discovered what its function is or should be.

The Veterans' Hospital Dilemma

Most people assume that the main function of the VA system is to provide medical care for veterans suffering from war casualties, but the fact is that only 15% of the cases are service-connected, and even those are not well handled for several reasons. For one thing,

the VA hospitals are not conveniently located; in some cases they are
hundreds of miles away from the residence (if any) of the veterans
suffering from disease, drug addiction, or amputation or a combination of these afflictions. It is too far away for the veteran or his family
(once more—if any) to utilize conveniently; it is much easier and more
effective to rely on nonprofit county hospitals. This is true of the
general hospitals. The veterans' psychiatric hospitals, however, treat
a more stable group of patients on a long-term basis and perform far
more efficiently.

The Vietnam Veterans

There has been a profound change in the age and social composition of veterans since the conflict (not a declared war, of course) in
Vietnam. Unlike veterans in previous wars, the Vietnam veterans
were discharged, if honorably, after service in Vietnam for one year,
so that there was not a sudden flood of veterans, but a steady stream.
Because of the unpopularity of the war, the veterans were discouraged, mostly unemployed, frequently discriminated against for
being homeless, addicted to drugs, and generally unwelcome in their
communities. If they were admitted to VA hospitals, they found most
of the beds occupied by veterans of World War I and II, and most of
them were not receiving medical care, but were being housed, bedded,
and treated for life, like the patients in nursing homes. Rehabilitation was spotty or nonexistent.

To the younger Vietnam veterans, this was a disheartening
prospect. What they needed and wanted was medical treatment,
physical therapy, psychiatric care, educational training, employment
help, treatment to cope with service-induced drug addiction, and
hope. Not warehousing!

The VA hospitals provide little preventive care, hospitalization
when outpatient service is preferable, little opportunity for family
doctors to participate effectively because of distance, failure to distinguish between chronic and acute care, and a profusion of bureaucra-
tic red tape.

There are many unsavory aspects to the war in Vietnam. Consider the state of New Mexico; by U.S. census count, Hispanics made
up 27% of the population in 1970 but supplied 69% of all those
drafted—and accounted for 44% of combat deaths.[18]

The use of Agent Orange, used to destroy vegetation in an attempt to effect the starvation of the Vietnamese, poisoned not only

the Vietnamese, but American soldiers as well.[19] Although there has been no credible scientific denial of this fact, the U.S. government for years refused to pay reparations to American veterans. They, their families, and some children malformed because of the poison were refused medical treatment.

Fiscal Summary

For $12.2 billion per year, one is entitled to expect more than bed-rest for veterans. The cost to the country for the scandal of the veterans' hospitals can be seen in our expensive homeless problem, criminal addiction costs, expensive therapy for minor problems, poorly focused treatment goals, and the soaring expense of treating avoidable ills.

On May 20, 1990, the Department of Veterans Affairs of Veterans Health Services and Research Administration, Washington, D.C., sent me a study prepared by the Joint Commission on Accreditation of Healthcare Organizations of 158 VA medical centers accredited by the Joint Commission for the calendar years 1987 through 1989, comparing their performance with all other accredited hospitals in the same area. Using 100% as the highest attainable scores, the mean score for VA facilities was 69.8, while the mean score for all other hospitals was 77. Although it is not easy to gauge the waste here, it is clear that the performance of the VA facilities is roughly 10% (77 minus 69.8 = 7.2) worse than the performance of the non-VA facilities. If we look at Note 11 of the schedule of expense listed in the annual report for 1988 prepared by the Department of Veterans Affairs, we find that actual outlays included:[20]

	Millions
Medical care	$10,045
Medical and prosthetic research	197
Medical administration	40
Total	$10,282

Knowing that the performance is roughly 10% worse than the performance of other hospitals, we can assume a waste of roughly 10% of $10,282 million, or $1,028 million. From what I have said about the waste in the operation of non-VA hospitals, we can be justified in stating that the waste of VA hospitals was in excess of $1,028 million, or one billion dollars.

The table of highlights in the annual report referred to above is very impressive. There, it is under the heading "Home Care":

Comparative Highlights

Item	FY 1988	FY 1987	Percent Change
Facilities at end of year			
Medical centers—hospital care and outpatient care	172	172	N/A
Nursing home care units[1]	119	117	+1.7
Domiciliary care units[1]	27	16	+68.8
Independent or satellite clinics	60	56	+7.1
Independent domiciliary and clinic	1	1	N/A
Employment (full-time equivalent)	202,178	202,651	-0.2
Obligations (millions)	$10,540	$9,960	+5.8
Medical care	10,230	9,673	+5.8
Research in health care	215	210	+2.4
Medical administration and miscellaneous operating expenses	47	42	+11.9
Other medical programs	48	35	+37.1
Inpatients treated[2]	1,224,375	1,465,703	-16.5
VA facilities[2]	1,130,283	1,371,757	-17.6
Hospitals[2]	1,086,456	1,332,056	-18.4
Nursing homes	27,220	25,567	+6.5
Domiciliaries	16,607	14,134	+17.5
Other facilities	94,092	93,946	+0.2
Average daily inpatient census	95,673	97,442	-1.8
VA facilities	69,516	71,346	-2.6
Hospitals	52,111	54,564	-4.5
Nursing homes	11,344	10,945	+3.6
Domiciliaries	6,061	5,837	+3.8
Other facilities	26,157	26,096	+0.2
Outpatient medical visits[2]	23,232,895	21,634,757	+7.4
VA staff	21,473,403	19,837,424	+8.2
Fee basis	1,759,492	1,797,333	-2.1

[1] Located within VA Medical Centers.

[2] FY 1987 inpatient figures include 255,094 one-day dialysis treatments. Beginning with FY 1988, this workload is excluded from inpatient data and included in outpatient data.

The report proceeds to describe in glowing terms the VA's hospital care, ambulatory care, dentistry, geriatric research, care of patients with dementia, programs for homeless veterans, treatment, research, and education related to over 5,000 AIDS patients in 1988, health care for women veterans, housing assistance, drug abuse, severe post-traumatic stress disorder (PTSD), etc.

However, an American Legion task force in January 1990 reported:[21]

With the assistance of Department Service Officers, task force members conducted interviews with 101 veterans who have been denied care or discharged from VA medical centers because of budget problems. Here's what some of the veterans told the task force:

* One midwestern Vietnam veteran now has to travel 600 miles for treatment from a private rheumatologist since being cut off from care at the VA hospital in Sioux Falls, S.D.
* A 59-year-old Korean War veteran who received treatment for post-traumatic stress disorder at a VA hospital was denied further care. He was refused care at VA's Veterans Outreach Centers because by law they only can treat Vietnam veterans.
* A 74-year-old WW II veteran who claims to have suffered hand and leg injuries in combat in Guam and Okinawa is unable to prove his disability claim. He had been receiving regular VA health care but has since been denied care—another casualty of VA's ongoing fiscal woes. The veteran has no supplemental health insurance.

The following is an excerpt from an article in *Vietnam Reconsidered*:[22]

When I was drafted I weighed 185 pounds, and upon my return from Vietnam I weighed 143 pounds. The first symptom that I developed was numbness in the hands and feet; later I developed the skin growths; and at present I have nerve damage. I have had almost every type of test there is for Agent Orange. In 1981, I was a patient at the Philadelphia Veterans Administration hospital; a nerve biopsy was conducted on my right leg. The sural nerve was removed, and the results were that I have peripheral neuropathy and was informed that there is no way to determine how this will progress. So there is still no answer to my health problems and those of other Vietnam veterans.

The time is now, not ten or twenty years from now, to help the Vietnam veterans and their families. We are not asking for pity, but only to be treated fairly.

A congressionally mandated VA study conducted by Research Triangle Institute found that among all veterans' perceptions of VA and its services the following prevailed:[23]

* 51% were not aware of benefits available to Vietnam-era veterans.
* 67% would prefer to go to facilities other than VA in emergency situations.
* 37% said VA did not provide security and peace of mind for the needs of Vietnam veterans.
* 65% did not feel they were fully informed about the availability of Agent Orange examinations at VA facilities.

The reader, of course, is free to choose between the claims of the VA or the critical statements thereof.

Health Maintenance Organizations

The term health maintenance organizations (HMOs) is very impressive, but as currently used does not describe a single type of entity, but a number of widely disparate organizations. In reality it is a generic term, including group-practice HMOs, staff-based HMOs, nonprofit and proprietary HMOs, network, individual practice association (IPA) HMOs, etc.[24] Some of the health insurance companies are affiliated with or are in the process of becoming HMOs.

How It All Got Started

HMOs were the outgrowth of an experimental program established during the Depression in 1933.[25] The Los Angeles Aqueduct was being built in the desert and the workmen naturally needed health services. To provide that, Dr. Sidney R. Garfield established a small hospital on a fee-for-service basis, which, as it turned out, did not generate enough revenue for the physicians to make ends meet. Dr. Garfield, together with the aqueduct contractors, succeeded in having the insurance carrier pay him a percentage of the workers' compensation premium for the care of job-related injuries and set up a plan covering non-job-related health care services for a monthly rate per worker of $1.50, collected by payroll deduction.

This approach satisfied the physicians and the hospital, effectively spread the enrolled workers' risk, and provided a reasonable level of care. It also set the basis needed for planning and budgeting. Inspired by the success of this operation, Edgar J. Kaiser persuaded Dr. Garfield to set up a similar plan for the workers building the Grand Coulee Dam under Kaiser management in the state of Washington. It also extended the coverage to include the workers' families.

In 1942, Kaiser, with Dr. Garfield's help, established the same type of plan for shipyard and other workers, and toward the end of World War II, the plans were opened to communities and other industries. So successful was it that in November 1967, the National Advisory Commission on Health Manpower studied the Kaiser Permanente Medical Care Program (Kaiser Plan) and concluded that it "has achieved real economies, while maintaining high quality of care . . ."

The Structure of the Plan

The Kaiser Plan is decentralized, each of the regions managing its own operations. The Kaiser Foundation Health Plan, Inc., which is nonprofit, owns outpatient facilities, and contracts with Kaiser Foundation Hospitals to provide or arrange hospital services for its members and with a Permanente Medical Group to provide medical services to its members. Another entity is a Permanente Medical Group, which is either a partnership or professional corporation that provides medical services to its region. The regions cooperate with each other and sponsor charitable, educational, and research activities. By 1990 the combined 12 regional plans included 7,760 full-time physicians, 66,000 nonphysician personnel, 28 medical centers with nearly 7,000 licensed hospital beds, and over 200 outpatient medical office locations. The plans have over 6.5 million members nationwide. Total assets are valued at about $6.5 billion.

The Kaiser Plan claims it is capable of delivering health care services efficiently and economically because of a number of built-in positive factors, as follows:

- Because fees are prepaid, the doctors or the hospital have no incentive to perform unnecessary surgery or treatment. For example, if bypass heart surgery or tonsillectomy or Cesarean delivery are not medically required, the operation is not necessary.
- Physicians involved in the plan are able to devote themselves to their professional duties 100% without spending their expensive time doing bookkeeping, promotion and computer activities.
- Physicians are involved in rendering services that are medically necessary; they do not have to worry about enhancing their income by rendering service for optional procedures.
- The ratio of physicians to patients in the Kaiser Plan of Northern California is 1 to 725, as compared to the rest of the community where the ratio is 1 to 350 or 375. That means that the Kaiser physician service cost is substantially lower.
- Preventive service is encouraged so that there is early detection of disease, which makes early treatment possible, thus keeping the cost lower.
- Alcohol, drug abuse, tobacco abuse, and obesity clinics are made available, which can also reduce medical treatment costs.

The HMO Stampede

The success of the Kaiser Plan set the stage for a proliferation of organizations claiming to be HMOs. Because the definition was vague at best, if an organization helped in the delivery of health care services, who could prevent its calling itself an HMO? From its very inception, the United States has demonstrated remarkable flexibility in the use of definitions. In the Declaration of Independence, published on July 4, 1776, Thomas Jefferson wrote, "We hold these truths to be self-evident; that all men are created equal. . . ." Jefferson, of course, was a slave owner, and did not consider blacks part of the human race.

Let us first consider the term "health maintenance." Obviously, to maintain health you must start with a healthy person. You cannot maintain the health of a person with terminal cancer; at best you can prolong that person's life or alleviate suffering. Most HMOs will not allow persons with serious ailments or physical disabilities to enroll in their plans, and HMO members are either prepaying fees them-

selves or being covered by employers. Consequently, we are looking at
a population in better health and financially more affluent than the
population being cared for in county hospitals.

The Group Health Association of America, an HMO trade organization, as reported in the *San Francisco Chronicle,* May 8, 1991,
stated that the Bay Area of California has the largest concentration
of HMO users in the nation, the members allegedly constituting 46%
of the Bay Area population.[26]

The HMOs have a bewildering variety of plans, some having
deductibles,[27] some providing eyeglasses, some having special rates
for children, some having reduced rates for medicines, some having
their own hospital facilities while most do not. Throughout the
country there are more than 600 HMOs, including the various
regional branches of some national organizations. Large hospitals
have banded together to form HMOs for members of the community
who wish to enroll, and HMOs for enrollees over 65 years of age. As
there is more emphasis on planning by HMOs as compared to health
care providers in general, some reductions in health care service
costs are effected.

Summary

In spite of all the positive features, we cannot overlook the
fact that the HMOs, like other segments of our health system, have
a number of weaknesses. Some patients complain of long waiting
times for routine appointments, insufficient emphasis on preventive care, etc.

In addition, HMOs require prepayment beyond the reach of the
financially destitute minorities who have no health care coverage
whatever. And the prepaid fees keep rising year after year at a far
greater pace of inflation than occurs in the rest of our economy.

In my opinion, however, the most hopeful accomplishment of the
HMO development is that it has demonstrated that *planning and
budgeting are not only possible but can be somewhat effective in
controlling costs,* and that is what critics of any form of national
health insurance steadfastly deny.

As is the case in the private hospitals, county hospitals, nursing
homes, etc., the health care alternatives provide practically no care to
the indigent, children, minority groups, poor pregnant women, and so
forth. That never was their intention.

As stated in the *New York Times,* February 9, 1992, George Bush would solve our health care problem by cutting reimbursement out of Medicare and Medicaid (already inadequate—my words, not his) in unspecified amounts, proposing a cap on malpractice awards (how much also unspecified), and using the savings to buy health insurance for poor families. No health care expert in the country supports such a bombastic plan.

7. Mental Health Services and the Homeless

One of the most chaotic components of what is euphemistically referred to as the American health care system is the mental health care program. Part of the problem arises from the fact that the terms "mental health" and "mental illness" are not clearly understood by those who draft the laws, administer them, or treat the supposedly mentally ill. As defined in the constitution of the World Health Organization (WHO), "health is a state of complete physical, mental, and social well-being, and not merely the absence of disease or infirmity." The absence of disease or infirmity sounds pretty good to me as a layman, but if that is not clear, the World Federation for Mental Health notes that the concept of optimal mental health refers not to an absolute or ideal state but to the best possible state insofar as circumstances are alterable. That sounds something like "the best of all possible worlds" encountered by Dr. Pangloss in *Candide*, but as I recall, he did not find circumstances alterable. But let us move on to something more specific.

The Medical and Health Encyclopedia[1] breaks down functional mental disorders into four categories—neuroses, psychosomatic disorders, personality or character disorders, and psychoses. We shall discuss them briefly in that order.

Neuroses commonly display emotional rather than physical symptoms. The most common symptoms are anxiety, conversion, obsessive-compulsive, depressive, and phobic reactions.

Psychosomatic disorders (also termed psychophysical disorders) constitute a very large portion of the caseload of a general practitioner and are not caused by any organic disease. Though psychogenic in origin, they are nonetheless responsible for a great deal of suffering.

The personality or character disorders include passive-dependent reactions by individuals who need excessive emotional support, withdrawn schizoid people indifferent to others, paranoid persons suffering from feelings of persecution, and sociopaths lacking a sense of personal responsibility or of morality.

Psychoses differ from neuroses in that the psychotic individual displays a more complete disintegration and a loss of contact with the outside world. The most common form of psychosis is schizophrenia. Different types of schizophrenia, simple hebephrenic, catatonic, and paranoid, present varying stages of personality disintegration, paranoia, and withdrawal from reality. Bipolar illness, formerly known as manic-depression, is also a fairly common psychosis.

The list of disturbances we have described sounds as though it might well fill a roster of mental illnesses for any mental health care system, but unfortunately that is far from the complete story. We must of necessity include victims of drug abuse, alcohol abuse, child abuse, elderly people suffering from a variety of senile dementias, victims of AIDS dementia, patients with tertiary syphilis, prison inmates with disorders listed above, children maladjusted because of lack of adequate food, housing, and education. They come from broken homes or families ostracized for racial and ethnic reasons. Frequently their parents too have severe mental disorders. Because access to the state institutions is very limited, there is now no governmental provision for the care of developmentally disabled people. This imposes a very onerous burden on their families. Private nonprofit charitable organizations such as the Muscular Dystrophy Association and the Cerebral Palsy Association do what they can to help do what a decent health care system should bo doing. However, we, the general citizenry, pay in any case because we make charitable contributions and pay larger taxes to make up for the taxes not paid by the tax-exempt organizations.

The American Psychiatric Association publishes a very imposing *Diagnostic and Statistical Manual of Mental Disorders*. The latest edition is *DSM-IIIR*, approximately 500 pages in length, describing in bewildering detail every conceivable and inconceivable type of mental disorder. Some idea of what is included in this manual can be understood from the following extract:

300.1 Hysteria

Mental disorders in which motives, of which the patient seems unaware, produce either a restriction of the field of consciousness or disturbances of motor or sensory function which may seem to have psychological advantage or symbolic value. It may be characterized by conversion phenomena or dissociative phenomena. In the conversion form the chief or only symptoms consist of psychogenic disturbance of the function in some part of the body, e.g., paralysis, tremor, blindness, deafness, seizures. In the dissociative variety, the most prominent feature is the narrowing of the field of consciousness which seems to serve an unconscious purpose and is commonly accompanied or followed by a selective amnesia. There may be dramatic but essentially superficial changes of personality sometimes taking the form of a fugue [wandering state]. Behaviour may mimic psychosis or, rather, the patient's idea of psychosis.

As the manual states, the last decade has seen a growing recognition of the importance of diagnosis for both clinical practice and research. The manual facilitates those functions, and it is also very useful for insurance purposes, enabling the insurance companies and the practitioners to speak the same language if not for care and treatment purposes then at least for reimbursement purposes.

We have already discussed the role of hospitals in the United States before the discovery of anesthesia and other medical advances for the treatment of the physically ill. Because little effective care was available at that time, hospitals were mainly warehouses for the sick and a method of segregating them to protect the rest of the community from infection.

Similarly, individuals who, because of mental illness, were a danger or potential danger to themselves or others, were placed in so-called mental institutions commonly referred to as insane asylums. Because the federal government traditionally did not assume responsibility for the care of mental patients, each state ran its own program and, as might have been expected, the quality of care varied widely from state to state. In many cases the abuses were so heinous that they inspired reformers to write scathing polemics exposing them. One of the most effective was *The Snake Pit* by Mary Jane Ward in 1946 (it later became a successful motion picture). Another expose was *The Shame of the States* by Albert Deutsch in 1948.

In the United States, psychiatrists and psychoanalysts are, almost without exception, medical doctors, although Sigmund Freud, the great pioneer in the field, did not feel that a medical doctorate was a necessary prerequisite for the practice of psychiatry. The AMA and the American Psychiatric Association (APA) assumed that the treatment of mental illness was a medical problem and they were successful in taking control without any real opposition.

The fact is that a large portion of what we call mental illness results, as we have seen, from addictions, depressed economic status, discrimination, the aging process, and some mental illnesses for which there is no known cause or treatment at this time. Some drugs can control symptoms in certain cases, but there is no sensible reason, other than tradition, why only a medical doctor can prescribe them. In addition, it should be noted that the clientele of most psychiatrists consists of those who can afford high fees, so that many of the psychiatrists have little or no contact with members of the lower classes. Social workers, nurses, and psychologists have much more experience in this area.

After World War I, the treatment of certain types of mental disturbances really began. The use of drugs or chemicals was instituted; sodium amytal provided treatment for World War I soldiers suffering from shell shock. It offered a prolonged restful sleep, after which the patients could tolerate some form of psychotherapeutic treatment. In the 1930s, insulin shock therapy was tried but, because of serious brain damage to the patients, was soon discontinued. Electroshock therapy was used but the voltages were too high and, because the effects were only temporary and frequently harmful, its use diminished until now it is utilized only in low voltages to alleviate severe depression.

Certain drugs such as Valium and Prozac are widely prescribed by physicians of all kinds, for conditions ranging from genuine neuroses to life dissatisfactions of all descriptions, including what used to be called "the vapors" in Victorian novels. They are a virtual bonanza for pharmaceutical companies. Other drugs such as lithium, Mellaril, Stelazine, and Haldol, have been prescribed to control psychotic symptoms and enable the patients to function on some level in the community.

However, in recent years the original enthusiasm associated with these antipsychotic drugs has become somewhat tempered. It has been discovered that their prolonged use frequently causes severe side effects such as irreversible tardive dyskinesia, which takes the form of uncontrollable movements of the tongue, lips, hands, and even the entire body. It thus creates intolerable social problems and usually prevents the patient from gaining or holding needed employment.

World War II became a turning point for the health care system of this country. In Chapter 1 we discussed the Hill-Burton Act, which was intended to modernize health facilities and provide medical services to the indigent. It was very important even though it was not enforced for 25 years, and then only partially so.

The mental health system too was the subject of widespread

criticism, resulting in serious federal attempts to make substantive improvements. One of the more important determinants was the role played by conscientious objectors, or "conchies," as they were called popularly. During World War II, 30,000 of them who, for religious or other reasons, refused to be drafted into the armed forces, were assigned to serve as aides and attendants in a number of state mental hospitals. Some of them wrote horrifying articles on conditions they had observed, and although their reports were discounted at first, in time they were regarded more seriously. The following excerpt is taken from the book *Nowhere to Go* by E. Fuller Torrey, M.D.:[2]

He opened the door to another room. I stood frozen at what I saw. Here were two hundred and fifty men—all of them completely naked—standing about the walls of the most dismal room I have ever seen. There was no furniture of any kind. Patients squatted on the damp floor or perched on the window seats. Some of them huddled together in corners like wild animals. Others wandered about the room picking up bits of filth and playing with it.

Near my feet was a little old man trying to shine my shoes. He had stepped in some of the human excrement and it was oozing out between his toes. A patient was eating some food from a tray which had been placed on the floor beside a urinal into which a patient had recently defecated.

The Flickering Light

With such documentation, it was not difficult to convince some legislators to hold hearings that eventually led to significant actions intended to improve conditions. The seriousness of the situation was also emphasized by Dr. Thomas Parran, the surgeon general.[3] He reported in 1945 that half of all the hospital beds in the country, some 600,000, were occupied by mental patients.

Until 1940, private foundations and universities financed research in the United States.[4] In July, 1941, the Office of Scientific Research and Development (OSRD) was created, followed by the Committee of Medical Research (CMR) and a number of other related organizations on a national scale. The federal government, which, as we have seen, had left the problem to the several states, was now entering the scene.

Another development that caused a dramatic change in the

status of the mentally ill in the United States occurred in the last couple of decades. The inclusion of Medicaid (Title XIX) of the Social Security Act in 1965 made it possible to pay for the care of the mentally ill who were over 65 years of age in nursing homes. About 10 years later the Supplemental Security Income (SSI) program provided for monthly payments ($447 in California in 1984) to blind or disabled persons of any age if they had no or very little income or assets. Many political leaders in various states saw these two programs as a way to reduce the costs of operating state mental hospitals. These political leaders began a systematic process of discharging patients, rationalizing this patient dumping as a salutary method of returning them to treatment facilities "in the community." The discharge was drastic indeed. According to Rockville, Maryland, National Institute of Mental Health (NIMH), the number of patients in mental institutions decreased from 552,000 in 1955[5] to 118,000 in 1984,[6] a decrease of 434,000 or 79%.

One question, of course, is where did the patients go after discharge from state mental institutions? The answer to that is that most of them are probably dead by now, a few may have remained in the institutions, and the rest went to homes of relatives, halfway houses, prisons, and the streets. The important question, however, is where did the new mentally disturbed people go once access to the state hospitals was drastically reduced? This will be answered as I continue this discussion.

In November 1986, the director of NIMH testified before Senator Lowell P. Weicker's Subcommittee of the Committee on Appropriations regarding the neglect of the seriously mentally ill. He presented a chart illustrating how little is known about their care. The tabulation follows:[7]

	Number	Percent
Nursing home care	73,500	5%
State mental hospital care	104,800	6%
Short-time inpatient care	225,400	14%
Outpatient care	269,000	17%
Unknown	937,300	58%
Totals	1,610,000	100%

If almost one million individuals with serious mental illness have been lost to view, somehow our program must be in a sorry state indeed!

Before proceeding further, it will be helpful if we understand more of the dimensions of the problem and how the federal government proposed to deal with it after it had become obvious that the states had failed miserably.

The *U.S. News and World Report,* in its issue of April 24, 1989, stated that it has been estimated that there are two million Americans with disabling mental illness, and that 60% of them live with their families at least part of the time. Hundreds of thousands more reside in nursing homes and privately owned "board and care homes." Still others are in prisons and in and out of acute care hospitals. Some receive assistance from community treatment centers set up by the Community Mental Health Center Act of 1963. Unfortunately, many, many more are homeless. Early planners of community health centers envisioned the establishment of 2,000 community treatment centers, but fewer than half opened.

Now that we have described the dimensions of the problem and where the patients go, it is time to consider what happens to them when they reach their several destinations. Those living with their families, although they may have somewhat warmer relationships than the other victims, frequently lack adequate care because of lack of knowledge and skills of their relatives. They also can cause economic and emotional burdens for those who are trying to help.

The mentally ill persons who are eligible for Medicaid and who go to nursing homes usually fare badly because of the shortage of properly trained personnel to care for them. In many cases it is simply a case of warehousing, and an extremely expensive form of warehousing at that. Those who go to the board and care homes are in even worse shape because the homes are completely outside the governmental regulatory system and are not supervised in any meaningful way. Mentally ill prison inmates may receive minimal counseling, but a penal system such as ours, based as it is on punishment rather than rehabilitation, can hardly be expected to, and certainly does not, provide the sensitive care those inmates need. The acute care hospitals are not anxious to admit them because they prefer patients who pay larger fees. The mentally ill patients are discharged expeditiously once the crisis is over.

The ones supposed to be cared for by the community health centers encounter a number of difficulties that militate against effective treatment. In addition there is a very poor utilization of funds. The following statements explain these two assertions.

• Being poorly motivated, the patients frequently neglect to

keep their appointments, and because there is little follow-up, many stop taking needed medication and, as a result, relapse into their previous ill state. There are recent indications that sudden termination of certain types of medication, in addition to causing relapses, may precipitate new violent disturbances.
* When releasing patients, the institutions do not always make adequate housing or outpatient treatment available.
* The mentally ill often suffer from other physical illnesses, particularly if they are elderly. To disregard this, as sometimes happens, is one more example of compartmentalized stupidity that can result in severe suffering or even death.
* Some of the ex-patients, because of their poor adjustment, drug addiction, or inability to deal with sudden drug withdrawal, can and do commit violent crimes.
* Finally, the savings in many cases are illusory because a number of the victims need and get treatment intermittently or regularly in expensive hospitals.

Under the Bridges

Anatole France did not write that both the rich and the poor can sleep under the bridge. His statement was far more biting. He said:

The law, in its majestic equality, forbids the rich as well as the poor to sleep under bridges, to beg in the streets, and to steal bread.

This brings us to the final category, a shame and disgrace to our country—the homeless! The scope of the problem is scandalous although the dimensions are vague. The *Harvard Mental Health Letter,* Volume 7, Number 1, July 1990, stresses the following main concerns: Researchers have not been able to agree on a definition of homelessness. One definition is lack of regular access to a conventional dwelling. People who spend nights in a shelter and the rest of their time on the streets, in the parks, etc., are thus homeless. People in hospitals, jails, or nursing homes, with no friends or place to go when they leave, can be considered homeless. What about those who spend one or more nights or days in a shelter? What about those living alone in rat-infested hotel rooms? To cast these two questions in an ad hominem mode, would you, the reader, consider the last two categories homeless if either one were your lot? To count the homeless is difficult, if not impossible. They may sleep by day and wander by night or vice versa. They may deny that they are homeless to avoid assault, arrest, or confinement to mental hospitals. The National Coalition for the Homeless estimates a total of two to three million. The Department of Housing and Urban Development says 300,000. Take your choice. Several other characteristics of the relationship of the mentally ill to the homeless are mentioned in the *Harvard Medical Letter*. The homeless are no longer mainly middle-aged and older alcoholic men. The average age is now 35. Fifteen to 25% are women and a number of these women have children with them—they constitute 25% of the homeless population. Forty to 50% belong to minority groups. Ten to 40%, according to various surveys, suffer from severe chronic mental illness. Twenty to 30% are drug or alcohol abusers.

The *Harvard Medical Letter*, Volume 7, Number 2, August 1990, discusses the service available to the homeless. In essence, it consists of 5,400 emergency shelters. The number of people living in them, 180,000, is clearly a drop in the bucket. The shelters are the equivalent of the 19th-century almshouses; everyone agrees that they solve nothing but only postpone solutions. The following quotation describes them adequately, if devastatingly:

> The shelter is commonly a big room filled with rows of cots, beds or mattresses that accommodate 50 to 150 people. Many shelters provide showers or baths, meals, laundry facilities, clothing, and television; some also provide some informal counselling and referral. About half allow residents to stay during the day, and the rest turn them out in the morning; most require them to do some chores. Although basic needs are provided for, conditions in shelters can be as wretched as they were in some state hospitals 30 years ago. Many shelters are filthy, dangerous, and crime-ridden. Privacy is lacking and toilet facilities are often inadequate. Usually no one on the staff is trained to care for the mentally ill, who often avoid shelter because they are afraid of crime and violence, or simply cannot tolerate the crowds, noise, and confusion. Some have to be turned away because they would be too disruptive.

Then of course we have the hotel rooms: filthy, rat-infested, and claustrophobic.

And one step down, the street; under bridges, in doorways, parks, in the rain, snow, sleet, and garbage.

Peter H. Rossi reports that a Chicago homeless study in 1985 found that about one in four of the Chicago homeless had at least one episode in a psychiatric institution.[8] The Division of Mental Health, Substance Abuse, and Forensic Services of the Department of Public Health, City and County of San Francisco, in April 1990, published a *Strategic Plan for Mental Health, Substance, and Alcohol Abuse, and Forensic* [jail] *Services*. It compares the current system and an estimated adequate system as follows:

	Current Capacity	Estimated Capacity
Adult mental health clients	13,000/year	22,000/year
Geriatric mental clients	3,700/year	6,500/year
Abuse services clients	16,957/year	44,757/year

The plan sounds excellent, but the crucial question is unanswered. With San Francisco budget deficits and threats of budget allocation cuts for the treatment of the mentally ill, where will the funds come from to meet the estimated capacity expenditures? When I talked to the Deputy Director of Health for Mental, Substance Abuse and Forensic Services in September 1990, she said that no one knows.

According to the *New York Times*, April 15, 1990, of the 15,559 psychiatric beds available in January 1990 in New York, 14,000 are to remain next year. However, Dr. Irene Levine, the program director for the homeless mentally ill at National Institute of Mental Health, says, "the spigot is still not turned off. Mentally ill people are still becoming homeless."

Let us now look at the waste of time, effort, and money resulting from what we have been discussing. The funds spent to establish and maintain the community mental health centers are largely wasted because the centers do not reach the mentally ill, or only peripherally so. The state mental health institutions, by operating on a short-term emergency basis, force the mentally ill into nursing homes and acute care hospitals, which are very expensive whether the bills are paid by individuals or other third-party payers.

Recently I visited a mental health care facility in Belmont, California. A tour of the building and grounds and a discussion with an administrator about the possible admission of my (nonexistent) suicidal granddaughter whose parents can afford institutionalization for the treatment of her mental illness elicited the following information:

The hospital is modern, attractive, well-landscaped, and can accommodate 84 patients—12 children, 17 teenagers, and 55 adults. It is licensed by the California State Department of Health and appropriately accredited. It offers free educational services in the community and provides psychiatric, nursing, social work, dietary, pharmaceutical, testing, physical therapy services, etc., for the patients. It also operates an outpatient clinic.

When I asked what the cost of the program for my granddaughter would be, I was told, "$1,000."

"$1,000?" I asked.

The response was, "Yes. $1,000 per day."

The hospital's gross revenue is not too difficult to compute. $1,000 times 360 days amounts to $360,000 a year per patient; $360,000 times 84 (number of patients) equals $30 million plus. Let us assume that collections are not too good and that only $20 million is collected. If we estimate labor costs at $5 million (very liberal), and other costs at another $5 million (also very liberal), we end up with a net profit of $10 million, or 100% on cost. Whoever pays, whether insurance companies, Medicare, Medicaid, employers of the patients, or the patients themselves, and in whatever proportions, the cost is clearly excessive. And the partners or stockholders, whoever they may be, and whether or not they are the psychiatrists, are doing extremely well indeed.

I also visited the Menninger Mental Health Resource operated by a hospital in Burlingame, California. They offer what we may term a bargain basement price of only $500 to $700 per day.

Those who end up in the jails and become wards of the state are far more expensive to care for than if they had been treated more sensibly in the first place, and had been granted appropriate education and employment possibilities. In many cases health professionals such as social workers, marriage and family counselors, and psychologists can do as effective or even a better job than the higher priced psychiatrists. However, the state medical associations have fought consistently against licenses authorizing the practice of therapy by nonmedical personnel and their reimbursement by insurance companies.

The government should spend more money on research to determine possible genetic causes of mental illness. In the long run we might save funds by finding new methods of treatment. The community mental health centers are a waste of time and money because they are functioning at an abysmal level.

Our government practically ignores the prevention of mental illness and as a result we often face the far more expensive and ineffective task of trying to cure the full-fledged disorders. The procedure of instituting budget cuts for services to the mentally ill should cease to be a knee-jerk reaction every time a deficit appears on the horizon, because the budget cuts immediately exacerbate the problem and lead to further cuts in service.

In conclusion, we may say that much of the money spent on our mental health program is being poured down a bottomless rathole.

8. Waste, Fraud, and Abuse

It should be understood that some of the deficiencies described in this chapter, "Waste, Fraud, and Abuse," and the following chapter, "Preventive Medicine," are outside the health care arena. The National Health Insurance Program cannot eliminate the problems, but can alleviate them. This will be covered in the "Conclusion."

Fraud can be defined as an act of trickery or deceit and as used here involves criminal misrepresentation resulting in monetary gain to the perpetrator. Abuse may be misuse that is similar to fraud or it may result from ignorance of proper use. Waste is useless or profitless consumption or expenditure. However, although they may differ from each other, from the point of view of health care services, they have one thing in common—they contribute mightily to runaway inflation. And they share that dubious distinction with the phenomenon we shall discuss in the following chapter, the lack of preventive medicine.

What Price Administration?

It is undeniable that an efficient health care system requires careful administration but careful is not synonymous with extravagant. In the *New England Journal of Medicine,* on May 2, 1991,[1] there is an article entitled "The Deteriorating Administrative Efficiency of the U.S. Health Care System." Although Britain is mentioned in passing, the conclusions are drawn from a meticulous comparison of administrative costs in Canada and the U.S. for 1987. Some of the main findings are as follows:

- Insurance Overhead
  In 1987, insurance firms in the U.S. retained $18.7 billion for administration and profits out of total premium revenues of $157.5 billion. That translates to overhead costs of 11.9% as compared to 3.2% for Medicare and Medicaid. Together, ad-

ministration of private and public insurance programs consumed 5.1% of the $500.3 billion spent for health care, or $106 per capita. The total cost in Canada consumed 1.2% of health care spending, or $17 per capita.

- In the U.S., by using the same approach, the article concludes that for 1987–1988, hospital administration expenditures were $39.3 billion, or $162 per capita, whereas in Canada, the comparable expenditures were $14.14 billion, or $50 per capita.
- Nursing home administration expenditures in the U.S. were $6.4 billion, or $26 per capita; in Canada the comparable figures were total administrative expenditures $1.69 billion, or $9 per capita.
- Two rather complicated methods of calculation were utilized for physicians' billing expenses, but they are included in this table.

Cost of Health Care Administration in the United States and Canada, 1987

COST CATEGORY	SPENDING PER CAPITA*	
	U.S.	Canada
Insurance administration	106	17
Hospital administration	162	50
Nursing home administration	26	9
Physicians' overhead and billing expenses		
Expense-based estimate	203	80
Personnel-based estimate	106	41
Total costs of health care administration**		
High estimate	497	156
Low estimate	400	117

* All costs are expressed in U.S. dollars.
** The high estimate incorporates physicians' administrative costs derived by the expense-based method, and the low estimate costs derived by the personnel-based method.

All of this may sound terribly confusing and technical, but let us simplify the presentation. The United States population in 1987 was stated in the article as 243,934,000 people. If we could reduce our administrative expenditures to match Canada's, here is what we would have:

High estimate:

U.S. expenditures per capita	$497
Canada expenditures per capita	<u>156</u>
Possible savings per capita	$<u>341</u>
Total savings $341 x 243,934,000 people	$83.182 billion

Low estimate:

U.S. expenditures per capita	$400
Canada expenditures per capita	<u>117</u>
Possible savings per capita	$<u>283</u>
Total savings $341 x 243,934,000 people	$69.033 billion

It may not be possible to match Canada completely, but when we are talking about *possible savings of $69 billion or $83 billion,* it is certainly worth our best shot.

The article concludes with a dire prediction:

The house of medicine is host to a growing array of specialists in fields unconnected to healing. At its present rate of growth, administration will consume a third of spending on health care 12 years hence, and half of the health care budget in the year 2020.

If one should assume the premise that higher administration costs ensure better health care, let us refer to a *Health Management Quarterly* survey reported in the first quarter of 1989. I shall mention a few of the findings here. Exhibit 1 compares the health systems of the U.S., Canada, and Great Britain (G.B.):

Exhibit 1
Three Health Systems: Comparative Facts at a Fingertip

Type of system	United States Mixed private/public	Canada Government insurance	Great Britain National health service
Population (in thousands)	240,856	25,625	56,458
Per-capita health spending	$1,926	$1,370	$711
Health as % of GNP	11.1%	8.5%	6.2%
Life expectancy, 1985 (years at birth)	74.7	76.5	74.8
Infant mortality, 1985 (rate per 1,000 births)	10.6	7.9	9.4

Data are from 1986 unless otherwise noted.

Information on Exhibits 3 and 4:

	Satisfaction with Hospital Stay			Satisfaction with Doctor Visit		
	U.S.	Canada	G.B.	U.S.	Canada	G.B.
Very satisfied	57%	71%	67%	54%	73%	63%
Somewhat satisfied	28%	18%	22%	32%	21%	26%
Somewhat dissatisfied	7%	5%	8%	7%	4%	7%
Very dissatisfied	8%	5%	2%	6%	2%	3%

And finally, preferences for an alternative health system were expressed in Exhibit 5, condensed as follows:

Prefer U.S. system vs. G.B. system	68%
Prefer G.B. system vs. U.S. system	29%
Undecided	3%
Prefer U.S. system vs. Canada system	37%
Prefer Canada system vs. U.S. system	61%
Undecided	2%

From these tabulations, it seems clear that Americans are not convinced that we have the best possible health care system.

Before dealing with fraud and abuse, I wish to make a few introductory remarks. When I express criticism of some doctors, hospitals, nursing homes, etc., that does not indicate that I condemn them all; many adhere to admirable professional standards. For example, a number of physicians are aware of the shortcomings of our medical care system, are in favor of reforming it, and are examining systems in other countries in an effort to find remedies. As a proof of this assertion, I am including as an Appendix a list of articles for the last 18 months appearing in *The New England Journal of Medicine,* one of the most prestigious medical journals in the world. Additionally, when fraud and abuse in Medicaid are considered, you have to impinge on other fields as well, such as physicians, dentists, nursing homes, etc., because as the popular ditty puts it, "The knee is connected to the thigh bone . . . etc."

Medicaid Fraud and Abuse

The Department of Health, Education and Welfare (HEW), under the terms of the Freedom of Information Act, issued a list to the news media of physicians in individual practice who received more than $100,000 from Medicaid during calendar year 1974. The amounts ranged from about $100,000 to $792,266. HEW in the accompanying press released stated that "the fact that these physicians received the stated amounts should not be construed as any evidence of wrongdoing, nor do the amounts listed necessarily represent 'earnings' or 'profits.'" There are more than 300 names on the list. I have no knowledge as to the completeness of the list, or whether wrongdoing may have been involved in some of these cases. As we proceed with this discussion the reader can form his own conclusions. What makes these figures staggering is the comments we frequently hear from doctors that the usual Medicaid reimbursement rate is abysmally low.

The list referred to appears as an appendix in a staff report prepared for the Subcommittee on Long-Term Care of the Special Committee on Aging, United States Senate, U.S. Government Printing Office, Washington, D.C., 1976. Much of the following information has been extracted from that report (Staff Report). In 1975, $14 billion in Medicaid funds were paid to hospitals, nursing homes, physicians and other providers of service.[2] New York received 23.3% of those funds, California 12.4%, and Illinois 6%. Lesser amounts went to the remaining states. The payments have steadily mounted since then. A great deal of the fraud and abuse takes place in "Medicaid mills," a term used to describe unregulated, unlicensed facilities, generally located in run-down sections of large cities, many in stores with or without windows. Usually there are signs in the neighborhood directing prospective patients to the facilities. The staff report was compiled as the result of investigating major governmental reports, both federal and state, evaluating vendors' statements, interviewing public officials and physicians, evaluating questionnaires, having staff members pose as Medicaid beneficiaries, visiting facilities for treatment, and utilizing a number of other investigative techniques.

The staff report states:

The abuses most frequent in Medicaid mills are ping-ponging, ganging, upgrading, steering, and billing for services not rendered.

- "Ping-Ponging" is the expression given the most common mill abuse, the referral of patients from one practitioner to another within the facility, even though medically there is no need. Generally, patients come to see a GP or the internists—inter-

nists are particularly prized by mill owners. They command
the highest fees for services, attract the most patients, and
give the most referrals. Once the patient has seen the inter-
nist, reasons can be found for sending him or her to other
providers in the facility.
- "Ganging" refers to the practice of billing for multiple service
to members of the same family on the same day. It generally
occurs when one member of a family is accompanied in his
visit to see the doctor by other members of the family—most
commonly a mother and her children. The abuse occurs when
the physician or other provider takes advantage of their
presence and treats them without a specific complaint, or bills
as though he has treated them.
- "Upgrading" is the practice of billing for a service more extensive than that actually provided. A physician may treat a
suspected cold, for example, and bill for treating acute
bronchitis and laryngitis.
- "Steering" is the directing of a patient to a particular pharmacy by a physician or anyone else in the medical center. It is
a violation of the patient's freedom of choice.
- "Billing for services not rendered" consists of either adding
services not performed onto an invoice carrying legitimate
billings or submitting a totally fraudulent billing for a patient
the doctor has never seen and/or an ailment he has not
treated.

Other abuses include:

- Billing for work performed by others or by unlicensed prac-
titioners;
- Making multiple copies of Medicaid cards, apparently for mul-
tiple billing;
- Soliciting, offering, or receiving kickbacks;
- Billing twice (or more) for the same service;
- Billing both Medicare and Medicaid for the same service.

Two police officers were recruited to assist members of the staff
in making visits to the Medicaid mills. They were told to say "I think
I have a cold." All were examined by a doctor before making visits to
determine that they were in good health.

There is no way to get an overall description of the scam without
quoting from the staff report in some detail.

In the three months of our shopping activity in four states (New York, California, Michigan, and New Jersey), our investigators (perfectly healthy) were told the following:

(1) Private Roberts entered Gouverneur Medical Center in the Lower East Side of Manhattan, New York City, complaining of burning and discharge in his urinary tract. He was given a general physical and a tuberculosis (TB) test, told he had a heart murmur, and given an electrocardiogram (EKG). A second shopper, Investigator William Halamandaris, entered the same clinic several minutes later complaining of a possible head cold. His "head cold" was diagnosed as "sinusitis," he was given a general physical, and EKG, a TB test, told he had a severe heart murmur, and that he probably had rheumatic fever as a child. In addition, the doctor ordered a series of X-rays of the patient's sinuses and chest, and referred him to a heart specialist—all in the space of three minutes.

Third shopper, Patricia G. Oriol, chief clerk of the Senate Subcommittee on Aging, entered this same clinic a month later complaining of a possible cold. She was told she had a severe heart murmur and high blood pressure and told to return for further tests.

All three shoppers were given a large amount of medication and specifically instructed to have the prescriptions filled "at the pharmacy next door." (It is a violation of New York State law and federal regulations to refer a patient to a specific pharmacy.)

(2) At the Avenue C Medical Center, Darrell McDew, complaining of slight dizziness, received a general physical and was referred to the chiropractor and optometrist. He was given an EKG, scheduled for laboratory work, and offered a Vitamin B1 shot. As a result of his visit to the optometrist, Private McDew, who has 20/20 vision, received a set of eyeglasses (one of three pairs he received while shopping Medicaid mills). Private Roberts, entering the same clinic, again complaining of a urinary problem, received a general physical, and was referred to a chiropractor, optometrist, and dentist. Private Roberts also received a set of eyeglasses and was scheduled to return for extensive blood tests. Roberts was told to fill his prescriptions at the adjoining pharmacy.

(3) At the Riis-Wald Medical Center, one block away from the Avenue C Clinic on the Lower East Side, Private McDew was

given a general physical, referred to the chiropractor and the podiatrist. The podiatrist informed Private McDew that he had hammertoe and flat feet (for which the podiatrist placed "arches"—actually they were small pieces of felt—in his tennis shoes). He was also told that his feet sweat. Subsequently, the same shopper met the same podiatrist (again on referral as a result of a "Ping-Pong") in a second clinic in Uptown Harlem. The podiatrist, after putting face and name together, checked his notebook and informed our investigator: "Remember what you had before? Well, you've got it again." He placed another set of "arch supports"—this time in the investigator's oxfords. In addition to arch supports, Private McDew received skull and chest X-rays (more than 10) and was ordered to return "next week" for additional tests. When Private Roberts entered the Riis-Wald Clinic, he received a general physical and was referred to the chiropractor, who ordered a full set of X-rays. He was also referred to the podiatrist, but had to refuse treatment because his toes had been painted the previous day by another podiatrist.

(4) At the East Harlem Medical Center, Private McDew asked to see a podiatrist. He was sent, instead, to the general practitioner and owner. The doctor listened to his chest and referred him to the chiropractor. He saw the podiatrist only after he had seen all other practitioners in the facility. Despite the nature of his complaint, "The bottom of my feet hurt," blood and urine samples were taken and his chest and feet were X-rayed. The podiatrist prescribed ankle braces, which Private McDew was told to obtain "down the street" from a particular supplier. He was specifically referred to the East 116th Street Pharmacy to fill three pharmaceutical prescriptions which included two antibiotics. Private Roberts entered this same clinic complaining of tiredness and received a general physical. He was referred to the podiatrist and given a future appointment to see the psychiatrist. Blood and urine samples were taken. His feet and chest were X-rayed and he was given two prescriptions which he was told to fill at the adjoining pharmacy.

(5) On May 20 at the Family Health Professionals Office on Second Avenue, Uptown New York City, Private Roberts saw a general practitioner and was referred to a dentist and a podiatrist, who diagnosed a bunion on his left foot. On the following day, May 21, at the Urban Medical Group, a clinic located on Third Avenue, Private Roberts, complaining of a cold,

had a general physical and was referred to the optometrist and a podiatrist, who examined his feet and also diagnosed a bunion, this time on his right foot. Roberts has no bunions on either foot.

My reactions to these examples range from amusement to admiration of American ingenuity, to amazement at HEW, which hesitates to construe practices like this as evidence of wrongdoing, to indignation at the brazen fleecing of the taxpayers.

There are many examples of abuses by various "health" practitioners. Some of my favorites are:

In 1972, a Brooklyn chiropractor billed for 12 visits in less than one month for a patient who denied ever seeing the physician. Another Brooklyn chiropractor was indicted earlier this year and charged with submitting billings for treating people who were dead, for men in prison, for people who have been homebound for more than five years, and for children under the age of five he had never seen.

A New York dentist recently developed a technique for getting around New York's requirement of prior approval for major dental work. Before he was discovered by authorities, he was drilling holes in perfect teeth and X-raying the teeth with the newly created cavities. The X-rays were kept to justify the fillings which the dentist then installed in the once-healthy teeth.

Earlier this year a Maryland dentist was charged with 74 counts of filing for Medicaid payments under false pretenses. In one instance, he claimed he had extracted 38 teeth from one patient. *The average adult has only 32 teeth.* He had been billing the Medicaid program for more than $200,000 a year.

A New York physician last year was charged with spending less than three hours a day in his office and yet billing the program for more than $150,000—a rate approaching one patient every two minutes.

A Port Washington, N.Y., podiatrist billed for seeing 50 or more patients a day, more than 15 beyond the established quality care line, billing for 60 toe jackets in one day (an average practitioner does about four), X-raying two-thirds of new patients (the guidelines are about 40%). In addition, the Department of Health determined that 90% of the castings performed were unnecessary.

The Illinois Department of Public Aid is so inefficient in

monitoring its payouts that five optometrists and two optical companies were able to collect $1,235.40 during a seven-month period for 55 visits to eye care specialists by a seven-member public aid family. The family says it never received the services or the glasses.

The report has 287 pages. I have exercised admirable restraint in limiting my quotations.

What we are talking about here is not simply the chicanery and enrichment of some greedy providers. We are talking about:

* Shoddy, inadequate, dangerous health care.
* The failure of federal, state, and other local governmental bodies to enforce laws and crack down on abuses, known and well documented for years.
* The shameful refusal of the American Medical Association and other professional organizations to police their own membership.
* The fact that "one of the primary causes, if not the primary cause, of the city's [New York] and state's fiscal crisis has been its mismanagement of the Medicaid program" in the opinion of the investigating committee that prepared this report.
* The fact that Medicaid service is being curtailed because of claims that recipients of Medicaid are fakers and are bankrupting the system when in reality the government is responsible for abrogating its enforcement responsibilities.

In retrospect, we may say that all of these cases are part of ancient history, and that things like that cannot happen now. But on July 9, 1991, there is a newspaper article in the *San Francisco Chronicle,* page A2. The headline reads "12 Indicted in Biggest Medical Fraud Case Ever." A federal indictment charges that 12 people, beginning in 1985, began to park mobile laboratories outside health clubs and offered people diagnostic tests that they said were free or covered by insurance. Using many fictitious corporate names, they promised customers medical examinations and tests for free or at nominal cost. The patients then assigned to the labs all rights to insurance payments. Bogus bills were then submitted to about 1,400 California insurance companies in the amount of approximately one billion dollars. It is not clear how much of this relates to Medicaid, but that is not really too significant. The American public is paying the insurance premiums, and the insurance company payments are part of our health care system cost. It is a case of colossal waste, because no medical benefits were received.

Hospital Fraud and Abuse

Fraud and abuse in Medicaid, some aspects of Medicare, nursing homes, and pharmaceuticals are flagrant, easily documented, and set forth in great detail in government publications. In the case of hospitals, the process is less evident, but nonetheless vicious and devastating. The most important reason for the hidden quality of the abuse results from the fact that hospital activities are subject to more stringent governmental regulation than other forms of medical facilities. The fraud and abuse in the case of hospitals is a matter of omission for the most part, rather than commission, although the latter is not entirely lacking.

We have seen, for example, how hospitals have accepted government grants (Hill-Burton) and have promised to provide free or below-cost service in return, and how for twenty-five years they ignored that requirement. To a large extent that is still true.

Many hospitals and other health care providers have received a nonprofit, charitable, tax-exempt status and have omitted charitable service. This, as I have already pointed out, is sanctioned by the government in its Internal Revenue Service regulations.

Although hospitals get discounts when purchasing drugs, they frequently do not pass those discounts on to the patients. Because a good many of these hospitals are nonprofit and exempt from tax, this practice constitutes a violation of their nonprofit status from a moral and perhaps legal point of view.

Until recently the hospitals' desire to increase occupancy led to unnecessarily lengthy stays in the hospitals. This was clearly evidenced by a comparison of the average length of patient occupancy in the normal hospital as compared to the health maintenance organizations. Of course this resulted in greater charges for Medicare reimbursement, as well as reimbursement from other insurance and patients themselves. This occurred while the cry was raised on all sides that medical costs were wildly inflationary.

As described in a previous chapter, Medicare has changed the method of reimbursement from retrospective to prospective in an effort to reduce costs. How the new system can harm patients is illustrated in an article written by Dr. F. Rahman, chief of hematology and oncology at Angelo Community Hospital, San Angelo, Texas.

Here are a few excerpts from that article, *San Francisco Chronicle,* January 25, 1986:

> A 65-year-old woman has been lying in the hospital for six weeks. She is suffering from complications of colon cancer—obstruction of the bowel, severe pain, nausea, and vomiting. She has a tube in her stomach and a urinary catheter. She is on morphine around the clock. Surgery has been futile. Her seven-year battle with cancer is finally near the end. But now she has also become the victim of Medicare rules—specifically, Diagnostically Related Groups (DRG).
>
> In the case of the 65-year-old woman, the diagnosis grouping allows her only 5.9 days of hospitalization and $1,865 worth of medical care. The hospital has already spent nine times that amount.
>
> So here I am, her physician, at a loss about what to do with her. She is unable to go home, the nursing home won't take her back, and she cannot stay in the hospital. Her case is not unique. In short, Medicare's payment system is not working. It puts doctors and hospitals in the position of denying crucial care or losing money.
>
> Although cutting costs has become popular, some facts must be made clear. An 85-year-old patient with diabetes, emphysema, heart disease, and pneumonia will take longer to recover than a younger patient who simply has pneumonia and is otherwise in good health. Yet, in the eyes of Medicare, both have the same diagnosis grouping, and the hospital is reimbursed the same amount.*

David Perlman, the science editor of the *San Francisco Chronicle,* in an article in that same paper, February 6, 1986, has an extended exposition on the same subject and concludes with this:

> The result, according to Carroll L. Estes, chief of the UC research team, is that hospitals are forced to move older patients out "sicker and quicker"—and into nursing homes and home health programs that can no longer provide adequate care be-

---

* Copyright © 1986 by the *San Francisco Chronicle.* Reprinted by permission.

cause of budget limitations.*

This is another example of how what seems to be a logical step in the direction of cutting costs may turn into a hospital abuse, aided and abetted by government bureaucracy.

Since patients are admitted to hospitals by doctors, a hospital usually attempts to provide all the equipment it can to attract doctors. This, in the past, has led to a number of wasteful procedures resulting in an excessive cost to patients and third-party pay sources. For example, several hospitals in the same area may each have expensive equipment utilized for only a small portion of the time. The item might be shared very easily at a greatly reduced cost. This would arise from lower depreciation and personnel costs, which could benefit the patient and third-party pay sources.

In an attempt to cope with this problem, governmental agencies have established a Certificate of Need program requiring a hospital to get approval before buying an expensive piece of equipment. The approval is based on adequate proof that the equipment is needed by the community and would not duplicate similar available equipment. But even this has been circumvented by a group of doctors together purchasing the equipment as a private corporation or partnership, which does not require a Certificate of Need, and placing the equipment adjacent to the hospital, which then pays for and uses it.

Another wasteful, inflationary procedure exists when several hospitals in the same area have underutilized departments, such as pediatrics or kidney dialysis centers, when one such center or centers could be shared by several hospitals at a much lower charge per patient.

One of the more disguised forms of abuse is the manner in which doctors enhance their own earnings by utilizing hospital resources and facilities financed by the public. There was a time when doctors had their own offices and paid for their own equipment. If doctors associated with hospitals do have their own offices now, they are usually small cubbyholes. Their real offices frequently are in the hospitals, and they own no equipment but use that of the hospital.

The accounting profession is in there pitching to "maximize" reimbursement, as they euphemistically term defeating cost containment. The General Accounting Office of the United States government as reported in an article in the *Wall Street Journal,* January 19, 1984, had this to say:

* Copyright © 1986 by the *San Francisco Chronicle.* Reprinted by permission.

When hospitals are sold and their assets revalued, the facilities can write off increased depreciation and interest expenses to Medicare, the agency said. However, the agency termed "questionable" the methods used by Hospital Corporation of America for Medicare cost reporting, saying they would tend to boost the amount of Medicare payments to hospitals. The agency said this would result in a similar rise in Medicaid payments because those disbursements are based on similar principles.

For the hospitals acquired by Hospital Corporation of America, capital costs rose $70.9 million in the first year after acquisition, while home-office costs were lowered by about $15.7 million, the agency said.

As a result, the agency said, the facilities had a net increase of $55.2 million in costs. The agency said the facilities are trying to charge those costs to Medicare.

These costs, the agency said, reflect an accounting change, rather than any significant upgrading in hospital facilities.

Hospital Corporation of America acquired IMA Corp.'s Hospital Affiliates International unit, including 54 hospitals, 18 nursing homes, and other corporate entities, for about $650 million in August 1981.

Medicare officials haven't decided how much of the increased capital costs they will allow, the agency said. A Gradison aide has said that the Ohio Republican asked for the GAO study after learning that Medicare costs rose $50 a bed at a Richmond, Va., hospital after its acquisition by Hospital Corporation of America.*

Hospitals, and the doctors associated with them, are wary of malpractice suits, order unnecessary tests, and, as former Health Secretary Joseph A. Califano Jr. claimed (as reported in an article in *The San Francisco Chronicle*), "We need more realistic standards of what constitutes careless conduct." As things stand now, the sky is the limit.

As I have mentioned before (it cannot be mentioned too often), another example of abuse is that private nonprofit hospitals are exempt from income tax, real estate taxes, etc., on the basis of their being charitable organizations. In fact, that is a gigantic fraud. They are conduits of profit—to doctors, banks, suppliers of drugs and equipment, accountants, lawyers, and whoever else can manage to

*Reprinted by permission of the *Wall Street Journal*, Copyright © 1984 Dow Jones & Company, Inc. All Rights Reserved Worldwide.

get his or her hands in the till.

During 1986, I was hospitalized for a short period of time in Mt. Zion Hospital in San Francisco. This is not an autobiography, so I shall not discuss the reason. While there, I had occasion to receive several drugs, theophylline (1 tab—200 mg), and castor oil (.2 fluid ounces). When I received the invoice from the hospital, the charges were $1.96 per tablet of theophylline, and $4.76 for each .2 fluid ounces of castor oil. The retail price at a local drug store in Belmont, California, was $.18 for the theophylline and $.09 for the castor oil. The charges can be compared as follows:

	Theophylline	**Castor Oil**
Charge by hospital	$1.96	$4.76
Cost at drug store	.18	.09
Difference	$1.78	$3.67
Profit	990%	4,080%

The assumption here is that the cost to the hospital is the drugstore's retail price, which, of course, is not true; the hospital's cost is much less.

Fortunately, because I was covered by Medicare, I did not have to pay those charges, but if I had not been so covered I would have been liable.

Charging 990% and 4,080% profit for a nurse to hand you a pill or a little container is flagrant profiteering.

Nursing Home Fraud and Abuse

Some subjects are so frightful to contemplate directly that sensitive, unperverted people have a tendency to look the other way in self-defense, or if they do look, they resort to irony when describing them. For example, there are three very good books analyzing some of the nursing home abuses. I refer here to *Too Old, Too Sick, Too Bad,* by Frank E. Moss and Val J. Halamandaris; *Tender Loving Greed,* by Mary Adelaide Mendelson; and *Unloving Care*, by Bruce C. Vladeck. The material in these books is immeasurably more horrifying than the titles.

Dante's *Divine Comedy* is termed a comedy not because it is humorous in the way we regard modern comedies, but because it does have a happy ending, proceeding from the Inferno to Purgatory to

Paradise. In one way it seems to describe nursing homes. In Canto III of *The Inferno,* we are told that on the gate to the entrance to Hell is the inscription "All hope abandon, ye who enter here!" That is appropriate, but there is a profound difference between what goes on in the *Inferno* and what transpires in some nursing homes. As in the Gilbert and Sullivan operetta, *The Mikado,* in the *Inferno* the intent is to make the punishment fit the crime.

To illustrate, in Canto XII, those who in life committed violence against others, such as Attila the Hun, Alexander the Great, and Rainier of Corneto (a notorious highwayman), were immersed in boiling blood. Whether or not you believe in this type of punishment, the intent is to provide a moral basis for it. But nursing homes partake of the characteristics not of the *Inferno,* but rather of Auschwitz.

The crime punished in Auschwitz was simply being a Jew. The crime punished in nursing homes is simply being old, poor, ailing, dying, a member of an ethnic or religious minority, or some combination of these.

We can get some understanding of nursing home fraud and abuse by answering several basic questions:

* How are nursing homes organized and staffed?
* To what extent are physicians involved?
* What are the most prevalent abuses?
* To what extent are nursing homes regulated?
* Has there been improvement in recent years?

How Are Nursing Homes Organized and Staffed?

As previously mentioned, in 1978, of the 18,722 nursing homes in the United States, 14,023, or 75%, were under profit control. And the industry was markedly successful in making profits. George Wells of the Federal Reserve Bank of Boston, in 1964 advised that profits after taxes commonly amounted to 10% or 20% of gross income.[3] Hearings conducted since then by various governmental agencies have confirmed the immense profitability of nursing homes. One of the reasons for the rosy profit picture is that, as contrasted with short-term acute care hospitals, nursing homes are staffed with poorly paid nurses' aides and orderlies. Where registered nurses are utilized they spend their time in supervising and administrative work, not in nursing. To put it more plainly, the personnel cost is low because the service is rendered by untrained employees.

To What Extent Are Physicians Involved?

Doctors practically ignore nursing homes for many reasons. Medical schools pay very little attention to geriatrics in the first place. It is also true that it is difficult to cure many ills of the elderly because of the irreversible aging process. Treatment lacks glamor. In response to a questionnaire from a Senate committee concerning geriatrics as taught in medical schools, Dean David Rogers of the Johns Hopkins University School of Medicine wrote:[4]

October 25, 1971
Senator Frank E. Moss
United States Senate
Washington, D.C. 20510

Dear Senator Moss:

I'm afraid, as with most medical schools, we do a thoroughly inadequate job in all the areas that you questioned me about. Despite being a member of a committee that examined a catastrophe in a nursing home here in Baltimore, the answer to all three of your questions is "no." More specifically:

1. No, we do not have geriatrics as a specialty in our curriculum.

2. We do not have programs in which students, interns or residents serve in nursing homes.

3. We have virtually no contact with the elderly who are in nursing homes—though we are currently exploring ways of developing some kind of program for students which will get them acquainted with the problems of the forgotten—our aging sick.

I firmly believe that all these areas are of increasing importance to us—and this school, as well as many others, should be involved in it.

Sincerely yours,
David Rodgers, M.D.
Dean of the Medical Faculty

The letter was franker than usual but the answers from other schools did not indicate a better approach to the problem.

In their efforts to distance themselves from nursing homes, physicians will prescribe medicines by telephone, will make so-called "gang visits," spending as little as one or two minutes with each patient, and then charging Medicare for a visit in each case.

In summation, it may be said that doctors rarely examine patients in nursing homes, often fail to report infectious diseases, and exercise little or no control over drug utilization.

What Are the Most Prevalent Abuses?

The litany of abuses staggers the imagination. Those most frequently encountered are improper use of drugs, negligence, lack of sanitation, poor meals, use of unnecessary physical restraints, theft of patients' funds, sadistic treatment, lack of fire prevention control, profiteering, kickbacks, and failure to provide supportive services such as eye care, dental care, etc.

The following illustrations have been taken from the book *Too Old, Too Sick, Too Bad**:

* In California, someone left a container of liquid Drano sitting next to a patient's bed. The patient drank it but did not receive medical attention for several hours. When she was taken to the hospital, eight hours later, emergency surgery was performed. She died about a week later from suffocation by ulceration and edema of the larynx.
* A woman's foot went unattended in another Chicago nursing home. Despite her daughter's repeated pleas for staff attention to her mother, she watched her mother's foot blacken and develop gangrene. It was finally amputated.

*Copyright by Aspen Publishers, Inc. Reprinted by permission.

- A patient left unattended in a Chicago nursing home was allowed to drink and smoke. She fell asleep, spilling liquor in her lap, and then dropped a lit cigarette. She became a human torch.
- A woman complained to the New York Health Department that her mother, who suffered from paralysis, was scalded by an aide trying to give her a bath. The patient died within a week.

The Senate Subcommittee on Long Term Care investigated the J. J. Kane Hospital, the second largest nursing home in the United States.[5] It is operated by Allegheny County in Pittsburgh, Pennsylvania. The following is verbatim testimony by employees of Kane Hospital:

Two male aides were struggling to pull a young multiple sclerosis patient out of bed into a wheelchair for an infrequent bath. "I'll take care of him myself," said one aide, slamming the patient into the chair. The patient groaned. The aide smiled at the patient and said, "You know I hate Dagos, don't you?" The patient was taken to a bathtub and sat quietly as the aide continued to berate him. "You know I hate you. Now that you are in the tub, I ought to drown you." The aide soaked a washcloth in the water and slapped the patient on the head and shoulders with it several times. "The headline in tomorrow morning's paper is going to read, 'Aide Kills Patient in Bathtub,' you Dago son of a bitch . . . " and slapped the patient with a wet washcloth again. This time the patient grabbed hold of the cloth. The aide punched him in the arm, forcing him to let go of the cloth, and decided that the bath was finished. The man, not wanting to be dropped, stiffened up as the aide lifted him out of the tub. He was punched in the stomach, pushed back in the wheelchair, hastily dried, and returned to his room.

The aide returned with another wheelchair patient to bathe. This was a black man, in his 70s and unable to walk. While undressing him for the bath, the aide discovered that the patient had a mild case of diarrhea. The aide lifted the man into the empty tub and began to spray him in the face with cold water from the sprayer used to clean out the tub after the baths. The man cried out, begging him to stop. The aide told him, "You better learn never to shit yourself again, nigger," and sprayed the man with cold water again. "Hey, watch him jump," said the aide to a colleague. He adjusted the sprayer so that a forceful half-inch of cold water came out, turned it on full, and sprayed the man's genitals. The patient screamed and covered his genitals with his hands. The aide whispered, "Do you know why I hate you? . . . cause you're a nigger." Holding the man's hands, the aide sprayed him again with cold water, this time the sprayer less than a foot away from the man's genitals. The aide then interrogated the man. "Are you a black man?" The patient did not respond. The aide (louder), "Are you a black man?"

"Yes," said the patient softly.

"Are you a nigger?" The patient did not reply. "Are you a nigger?" demanded the aide in a loud voice.

"Yes."

"Is this nigger ever going to shit again?"

"No," responded the patient weakly.

As the result of an undercover investigation of kickbacks between clinical laboratories and nursing homes in Chicago in 1976, Special Prosecutor Hynes estimated that half of the nursing homes in New York participated with suppliers in kickback abuses.

For documentation of the other types of abuse, I refer you to the book just mentioned.

To What Extent Are Nursing Homes Regulated?

Nursing home standards are set forth in "Conditions of Participation" for skilled nursing facilities in the Social Security Act and are amplified by detailed regulations. Seventeen conditions are considered.

If all nursing homes were to conform to them, nursing home health care would still be inadequate, but far better than it is. But in the world as we know it, one is reminded of the colloquy in Shakespeare's *King Henry IV*, Part I:

Glendower: I can call spirits from the vasty deep.
Hotspur: Why, so can I, or so can any man; But will they come when you do call for them?

In addition to the setting of conditions, there must be enforcement. And to return to the Bard, we may well say with Hamlet, "Ay, there's the rub." There it is indeed!

In spite of investigation by Ralph Nader and his task force, audits by the General Accounting Office critical of nursing home standards, the Senate subcommittee's investigations showing gross malfeasance, and many other investigations, only a very few nursing homes have been closed or fined. And this has been in an industry where all indications are that at least 50% of the nursing homes are substandard.

Has There Been Improvement in Recent Years?

In spite of vague statements that things are much better, little evidence has been produced to substantiate these claims. As reported in the *San Francisco Chronicle* of April 15, 1984, the same tired old horses that have been beaten for decades are still being beaten.

* The California Committee on Aging and Long-Term Care is considering remedial legislation to tighten regulation of nursing homes.
* Nine bills are being considered by the California Legislature to make it easier to protect patients in the 1,160 nursing homes in California.
* Heavier fines for malfeasance are being sought.
* Nursing home operators are a powerful group. This association has donated $414,128 to legislators and other state office candidates since 1981. Eleven members of the Aging Committee have received $26,023.

When this sort of meeting was held for the fiftieth time years ago, it may have been considered déjà vu. There is no respectable description for it in 1984.

The unfortunate truth is that when it comes to nursing home fraud and abuse, conditions have not improved in recent years. They have gotten worse. This has happened in spite of the valiant efforts of the Gray Panthers and other neighborhood public interest groups working for reform. And it has happened, to put it bluntly, because governmental enforcement has been completely lacking. And as usual we must emphasize that much of the money spent by patients, insurance companies, and governmental agencies has gone not for health care, but for excessive profits resulting from fraud and abuse.

Home Health Service Fraud and Abuse

Funds paid to providers of home health care for the poor and elderly in many cases have been diverted to the pockets of the providers. Some of this abuse is the result of poor government monitoring and enforcement of the laws and regulations governing the expenditure of such funds. Some of it is due to the greed and criminality of some providers.

In March 1977, two hearings were held before the Special Committee on Aging, United States Senate, in cooperation with the Subcommittee on Health and the Subcommittee on Oversight of the Ways and Means Committee, U.S. House of Representatives. The text of the hearings is published by the U.S. Government Printing Office, under the general heading of "Medicare and Medicaid Frauds."

A short explanation of how providers were reimbursed by Medicare for service to Home Health Medicare patients is in order here. Prior to the hearings the procedure had been as follows.

A Home Health Agency (HHA) billed the Medicare reimbursing entity for services rendered at an agreed-upon rate per hour or visit. The HHA would be paid on a more or less current basis. At the end of the HHA's fiscal year, the HHA submitted a cost report to the reimbursing entity. The costs included were those defined as "reasonable" in the rules and regulations of Medicare. If the "reasonable" costs exceeded the costs billed, Medicare owed the difference to the HHA. If the reverse was true, the HHA owed the difference to Medicare. The cost report was subject to audit by Medicare or an independent certified public accounting firm selected by Medicare.

The first case to be discussed here is the agency called the Home Kare Agency. Mr. Val Halamandaris, counsel for the committee, and other members of the committee, by questioning John Markin of the staff of the House Ways and Means Oversight Subcommittee, elicited the following facts:

Various corporations are associated with the parent corporation, Home Kare, Inc. The work performed by each is described in the list below:

Parent	Home Kare, Inc., a licensed Home Health Agency that provides nursing care and home health aide care. Medicare 96%, Medicaid 3%, commercial 1%.
Subsidiary	Flora's, Inc. The Showcase Beauty Salon.
Subsidiary	Unicare, Inc. Licensed Home Health Agency that provides homemaker service. For city welfare recipients 57%, commercial 43%.

Subsidiary	Flora M. Souza Therapy, Inc. Provides physical therapy services. Medicare 65%, Medicaid 3%, commercial 32%.
Subsidiary	Ambi-Care, Inc. Outpatient rehabilitation physical therapy clinic.
Subsidiary	Allied Paramedical Training Institute, Inc. Provides training to home health aides and homemakers.
Subsidiary	Health Care Legislative Council, Inc. Lobbying organization.

Mr. Markin listed some of the so-called reasonable expenses claimed on the cost reports submitted by the Home Kare Agency:

- A 450 SLC Mercedes Benz automobile driven by Flora M. Souza, president of Home Kare, Inc., costing $22,524, was being depreciated over four years and charged to Medicare and Medicaid.
- A 450 Mercedes Benz automobile driven by Jack Stewart, controller of Home Kare, Inc., was similarly charged.

Before being employed as Controller of Home Kare, Mr. Stewart had been an auditor with Travelers Insurance Company, the fiscal intermediary responsible for monitoring Medicare charges by Home Kare, Inc. As a matter of fact, he was Travelers' auditor in charge of the Home Kare accounts. The Mercedes was given to him one month prior to his leaving the insurance company. Conflict of interest could scarcely be more flagrant.

- Mr. Stewart in 1977 received about $43,000 in salary, and the company provided him with medical insurance, life insurance, and a pension fund, all at no cost to him. He also had an expense account.
- Mrs. Souza had three sisters and a daughter on the payroll; they had a leased Cadillac and a leased station wagon used only to go from home to the office and back. All of these are presented as reasonable costs.
- Mrs. Souza's combined salaries and compensation from the parent and subsidiary corporations amounted to about $145,000 for the fiscal year ended March 31, 1976.

Further testimony elicited some of the dirty tricks used to substantiate fictitious costs charged to Medicare. An invoice for two cheeseburgers, one hot dog, one roast beef sandwich, and three colas to go, $7.47, was changed to $47.47 and charged to business needs. A $43.40 meal expense, supposedly business, was paid for by Home Kare, submitted again on Flora Souza's business expense account as $220.00, and paid again as a business expense. Jewelry and clothing purchases by Flora Souza were disguised as business expense.

One must feel sorry for Senator Church, who at times seemed quite bewildered by the testimony. Take these two excerpts, for example:

Senator Church: So here is a case of glassware and the basket, personal purchases at a jewelry store, being charged to the government in the guise of meals expense.

Mr. Markin: That is correct. We also found a brass bed.

Senator Church: You also found what?

Mr. Markin: We also found a brass bed.

Senator Church: Brass beds?

Mr. Markin: Yes; there was a brass bed charged to one of the corporations. While at Home Kare we asked where that brass bed was and it was in Mrs. Souza's home. We also found other furniture purchases.

Senator Church: What about the beauty shop? That is not connected with medical care at all. I don't know of any Federal program that covers this beauty shop. Do you know about it?

How did the beauty shop expense get charged to the Government through the Medicare program?

Mr. Markin: I gave you the one example of the furniture. The Showcase—the beauty shop—bought the furniture at wholesale, sold it to Home Kare at close to retail and came out with a substantial profit? That is one example.

Then we have a situation when Mrs. Souza first wanted to get this corporation—The Showcase—going, and started by employing a beautician by the name of Kaye Bradley and paid her by Home Kare checks. Now when this was brought to the attention of the Home Kare people they said that she had been paid a total of about $8,500 of which they said about $5,500 of it was a mistake and the other approximately $3,000 was for training home health aides in proper hair care.

Senator Church: For proper hair care?

In the following excerpt the bookkeeper explains the simple method of falsification:

Mr. Halamandaris: Were you ever specifically instructed to falsify or to alter or to duplicate or to kite the expense sheets for Home Kare or any other corporations owned by Flora Souza? Were you given any specific instructions to do this; in other words, to represent that this was a luncheon attended by those people that you mentioned? Who told you to write that this was a meal attended by all these people?

Miss Harvey: Can we do one question at a time, please?

Mr. Halamandaris: Sure. Take any one that you are comfortable with.

Miss Harvey: Yes, I was told to write names and alter amounts on expense vouchers.

Mr. Halamandaris: Can you tell us who told you to do so?

Miss Harvey: I dealt mostly with Sharon Jack.

Mr. Halamandaris: Can you identify Sharon Jack, please?

Miss Harvey: She is Flora Souza's daughter.

Mr. Halamandaris: Did they do this with Flora's knowledge?

Miss Harvey: Did she do what?

Mr. Halamandaris: OK. Let me ask you this. Is it true that the money that was generated by double billing or by kiting and by writing out checks, which were endorsed by Flora Souza, was deposited to her account? Am I correct that you personally never benefitted from any of those checks that you wrote?

Miss Harvey: That is correct.

One of the more touching excerpts from the investigative memorandum submitted by Val J. Halamandaris and John Markin to the senators should gladden the hearts of all dog lovers:

Mr. V informed the subcommittee that the medical expenses for Souza's dog, Cherie, are written off to Medicare through Home Kare. Mr. A reports that Souza bought their dinner, and then ordered a $5.95 short rib dinner for Cherie. The whole thing was charged on American Express and likely to Medicare through Home Kare. Mr. B also asserts that Souza has purchased expensive food for her dog, also via American Express. (No verification.)

In addition to falsifying records, another way Home Kare defrauded the government and increased revenue was to pad the number of visits, listing visits that never took place.

After Mr. Stewart left Travelers, Mr. William Kenison was employed by them as senior Medicare representative, Medicare Part A. He testified that in attempting to audit Home Kare, Inc., he found that trial balances were out of balance as much as $600,000, that access to the books and records of related organizations was denied, and that, in essence, a proper audit was impossible. Flora Souza and Jack Stewart refused to answer questions, claiming protection under the Fifth Amendment to the Constitution. Flora Souza was sentenced to 18 months in jail and, having served her sentence, is now free.

The abuses in this case are obvious. The provider of service was fraudulent and criminal. Funds intended for service to the indigent were used to enrich the providers' owners. The governmental agencies displayed negligence, inefficiency, and callous disregard of their true enforcement obligations. The insurance companies and auditors failed in their public and professional responsibilities. The physicians exercised no control over the whole operation, although according to the special investigatory committee they were paid far more than comparable physicians in other home care agencies.

The day after the Senate subcommittee held the hearing on the Souza case, they held another on the case of Peter Gottheiner. Some of that testimony is preposterous.

The summary quoted from the appendix, investigative

memorandum prepared by Tom Cline, investigator, and Val J. Halamandaris, associate counsel, Senate Committee on Aging, presents the gist of the case, which I am summarizing as follows:

Peter Gottheiner was a provider of home health services for more than a decade, was suspended from Medicaid, and Medicare claimed that he owed $800,000 for unresolved audit exceptions. In spite of that, he continued to operate and still receive Title XX Social Security Act funds. He went into bankruptcy. However, he was still operating under a new corporate name, National Home Health Care, Inc. The summary also stated:

> On March 24, 1975, Mr. Thomas Tierney, Director of the Bureau of Health Insurance (BHI), wrote to the General Counsel of HEW indicating BHI's computation of audit exceptions and moneys owed to Medicare by Gottheiner's California Coordinated Health Care Service as follows:

Year	Overpayment
1967—audited cost report	$6,304.00
1968—audited cost report	76,320.00
1969—audited cost report	213,338.00
1970—failure to file cost report	449,522.00
1971—failure to file cost report	31,787.38
1971—current financing payments	69,000.00
Subtotal	846,271.38
Less claims held in escrow	41,616.32
Total indebtedness	$804,655.06

In spite of the mountain of evidence that flagrant fraud was being perpetrated, the government officials constantly stated that they had insufficient evidence to stop it. In my practice as a CPA, I have seen taxpayers who owe $32.50 in overlooked income taxes threatened by the Internal Revenue Service with attachment of bank accounts, etc. In the case of Gottheiner, the behavior of HEW personnel is not only incredible, it is scandalous!

Now a short excerpt outlining the role of the lawyers representing Peter Gottheiner. The person being interviewed is Frederick Keeley, a former employee of one of Gottheiner's corporations and a former employee of Flora Souza! The discussion at this juncture concerns an attempt on the part of Gottheiner to contract with the

State of Illinois to provide homemaker/chore services under Title XX of the Social Security Act.

Mr. Halamandaris: What further action was suggested in the memo? What route were they to take to secure the contract?

Mr. Keeley: It was suggested that the corporation continue to be in contact with those state officials and that an arrangement be made between a particular law firm in that state and the corporation.

Mr. Halamandaris: Is this a copy of the contract to which you refer?

Mr. Keeley: Yes, it is.

Mr. Halamandaris: That is a contract between the law firm and Mr. Gottheiner, is it not?

Mr. Keeley: Yes.

Mr. Halamandaris: Would you tell us, please, what the compensation is for the law firm in that contract?

Mr. Keeley: It is an attorney's contract between the Visiting Home Services and the law firm of Moriarty, Rose and Hultquist, Ltd. Under section 2 regarding retainer and contingent fees it indicates that the clients shall pay the attorneys a retainer fee of $7,000 in the following installments and it lists A through D and the installments. Later in that same document it indicates that on behalf of Visiting Home Services the attorneys will attempt to successfully negotiate contracts with the State of Illinois on behalf of the client and the compensation therefor will be 4.8% of the first million dollars in contracts and 1.2% of all sums in excess of $1 million.

Senator Church: The law firm's fee was to be based upon a percentage of the take?

Mr. Keeley: As it were.

Senator Church: As it were. The bigger the contract, the bigger the fee. Since they are talking about millions of dollars, that would come to a mighty tidy fee, wouldn't it?

Mr. Keeley: I imagine that it would, Senator.

Peter Gottheiner, unlike Flora Souza, did not invoke the protection of the Fifth Amendment of the Constitution. It is possible that he thought his testimony would be so confusing that nobody could understand it, and therefore he could not be found guilty of any misconduct or crime. It is also possible that his thought processes were as deficient as his moral sense. You can decide for yourself.

Representative Gibbons: Mr. Rostenkowski and I are going to have to start voting pretty soon and I certainly don't want to cut him off, but I want to ask him some questions.
Mr. Gottheiner, in 1973 through your home—did you charge $1,691 for pipe and tobacco costs?

Mr. Gottheiner: No, sir. I can explain.

Representative Gibbons: How did I get told you did if you didn't?

Mr. Gottheiner: All right; I made one mistake. Since I was the sole owner of the company, I had those checks made out on the company account, but they were debited to my income. In other words, I was the sole incorporator at that time of Health Help, Inc., and I figured—and apparently it was wrong—that is what started the ball rolling.

Representative Gibbons: How about the inaugural expense? Whose inauguration was that?

Mr. Gottheiner: President Nixon, and it was not an inaugural expense.

Representative Gibbons: $925. He was not inaugurated in 1975, was he?

Mr. Gottheiner: That was not 1975. The audit is 1973.

Representative Gibbons: Did you seek reimbursement?

Mr. Gottheiner: No, it was the same thing. I don't recall whether it was Congressman Burton. I met with someone, but anyway that was strictly my own business and I should have taken all the profit out and then paid it on my own, but it did not affect this in one way or the other.

Representative Gibbons: How about cash disbursements in 1973 for entertainment, $50,000.

Mr. Gottheiner: In 1973?

Representative Gibbons: Yes, sir.

Mr. Gottheiner: For which company? (Laughter.)

Representative Gibbons: You got me confused. I guess it is—

Mr. Gottheiner: No, I didn't ask the—

Representative Gibbons: It looks like $50,000.

Mr. Gottheiner: I did not ask the question to be funny.

Representative Gibbons: I understand.

Mr. Gottheiner: I wanted to tell you before I answer the question. In 1971 Visiting Home Services was formed and Visiting Home Services until 1973 had no contract, so probably the major part of it, because Visiting Home Services had no income, was charged, was regularly reimbursed by Home Services.

Representative Gibbons: But you sought reimbursement.

Mr. Gottheiner: Yes. Health Help was the only company who had a contract that was in business and they advanced money on many occasions, or I did, or the company for Visiting Home Services, until they got on their feet and for as long as I could keep it.

Representative Gibbons: Do you really need to entertain anybody that much?

Mr. Gottheiner: No, it was not entertaining, Mr. Gibbons.

Representative Gibbons: What was it?

Mr. Gottheiner: All right. We attempted to get contracts since 1972. There were a lot of travel expenses during the entire time of the existence of Visiting Home Services. Almost everything was billed on my credit card. When I went on a trip I then got that reimbursed. Both companies used my credit card regardless whether I traveled, whether other people traveled or whether I stayed at the motel or whether other people stayed at the motel.

Representative Gibbons: The staff writes this question that cash disbursements for entertainment according to the audit exceeded $50,000 for the period 1973. Either the audit is wrong or the staff is wrong. Now, who is wrong?

Mr. Gottheiner: If the audit picked it up as entertainment, then this staff was wrong. The staff was unfortunately wrong in a lot of things in the accounting department, but there was no way there was that entertainment. There was a lot of travel.

Gottheiner's model for testimony, I presume, had as its precedent the verses read by the White Rabbit to the jury in *Alice in Wonderland*. Here are the first two quatrains:

Alice's Evidence
They told me you had been to her
    And mentioned me to him:
She gave me a good character,
    But said I could not swim.

He sent them word I had not gone
    (We know it to be true):
If she should push the matter on,
    What would become of you?

That should be enough, but I cannot resist one more passage. Mr. Ralph P. Gomez referred to here was an employee of one of the corporations.

Senator Church: Well, I have no further questions.

Mr. Gottheiner: May I just make a couple more comments?
    On the other audit here for Mr. Manly, again for the record, on the last page I am referring to the audit of October 29, 1976, where, Senator, you have the compensation out of the other audit, but the figures as far as I am concerned are correct. I just would like to go briefly through the others because it is on my conscience to tell you.
    Mr. Gomez for the $49,000 he got, first of all, that was only for a 9-month period prorated over one or two hours a day where he made personal telephone calls. His hourly rate was $200 an hour. My daughter, Vivian, is listed with $1,875.

Senator Church: Mr. Gomez, what was he doing making telephone calls and getting $200 an hour for?

Mr. Gottheiner: What was he doing?

Senator Church: Yes.

Mr. Gottheiner: That is a question I asked myself a long time ago. (Laughter.)

Senator Church: The auditor indicates he didn't do anything.

Mr. Gottheiner: I think Mr. Gomez, if I may be very candid with you, should not be a case for the auditors.

Senator Church: Should not be what?

Mr. Gottheiner: Should not be case for the auditors.

Senator Church: Should not be case for the auditor?

Mr. Gottheiner: No; I think the category higher. I worked that hard for the company four years ago, I had a heart attack in a welfare office and to me, not even talking about financially, it was morally the worst blow when Mr. Gomez came in about one month later and I knew what was going to happen. I had, and I admit it, frankly, the worst crying spell and I tried to get drunk and get it over with, drink myself to death. I mean, I didn't do it, but I knew that Mr. Gomez was a wing of the company and that is not the first company.

But getting back to my daughter, $1,875; $375, the last check bounced. That made it $1,500 and that was charged to me.

My son was a full-time worker for the company and he deserved his income. The $8,300 from loan repayment he had to borrow once, and somebody gave him cash and wanted cash back and that was the transaction. There will be entries, there should have been entries, and I am sure there were entries for that money, for the $8,300. My ex-wife did some secretarial service, and the rest I charged. It was charged on me.

On May 3, 1983, six years after the hearing and over a decade after disclosure of the facts to the government, Peter Gottheiner surrendered himself to U.S. marshals to begin serving an 18-month prison term for signing a false statement in a financial transaction involving a $250,000 note.

According to an editorial comment in *Underwriters' Report*, published in San Francisco, December 22, 1983, Mr. Gottheiner has steadfastly maintained that he is innocent. He was scheduled for released in February from Terminal Island Prison in San Pedro, California, and intended to return to practice in San Francisco, where he has continued to maintain a physical therapy office.

Caveat emptor! In the immortal words of James Thurber: "Go east! Go east! The dam has broke!"

Lest you, the reader, assume that these two cases discussed in detail constitute exceptions, let me assure you that when unscrupulous operators know how lax enforcement really is, they utilize every trick in the book, and it's a very thick book with many, many pages. The obvious conclusion is that where enforcement is practically nonexistent, waste, fraud, and abuse ride high.

Pharmaceutical and Medical Test Fraud and Abuse

Chapter 5, on the subject of AIDS, includes a fairly comprehensive discussion of the excessive costs of AZT, the drug that materially helps AIDS patients. I shall not repeat it here except to say once again that the inflated charges constitute pure profiteering!

For thousands and thousands of years, people have experimented with drugs found in nature. In Genesis (9:20 and 21) we read that "Noah began to be an husbandman, and he planted a vineyard:

And he drank of the wine, and was drunken." The motivations for drug investigation and utilization have been many and varied. Alcohol, opium, cannabis, coca, coffee, tobacco, heroin, peyote, and many more drugs have been used for a variety of reasons by many cultures. Some of the reasons, whether successful or not, were the dulling of physical pain, enhancement of aesthetic experience, improved sexual performance and enjoyment, religious ecstasy, consciousness expansion, cure of physical disease, treatment of mental illness, and the search for thrills and excitement. In recent years with the development of science, to the list of drugs found in nature we have seen the emergence of synthetic drugs intended to perform specific functions.

When we refer to drug cultures we customarily think of addiction to narcotics such as cocaine, heroin, cigarettes, LSD, etc. The United States, according to the *Encyclopedia Britannica,* in the early 1970s, had approximately 120,000 drug addicts. The word *addict* is used loosely here to mean a person physically or psychologically dependent on a drug.

However, the United States is a drug culture in a more profound and frightening way. Dr. Milton Silverman and Dr. Philip R. Lee, in their book, *Pills, Profits, and Politics,* page 17, state the problem succinctly:

The total prescription drug bill for 1972 would thus be approximately $10.0 billion. To this may be added roughly $4.0 billion paid by the public for nonprescription or over-the-counter health products, giving a bill for all drugs of $14.0 billion. And finally, the cost of adverse drug reactions, estimated in 1971 to be at least $3.0 billion and now perhaps as much as $4.5 billion for hospital charges alone, should also be included in any aggregate appraisal of total drug costs. On this basis, the real annual drug bill to the public was at least $17.0 billion, or approximately 20 percent of all health care expenditures.

One of the most important things to realize about pharmaceuticals is that doctors in the United States have zealously and successfully reserved to themselves the legal right to prescribe drugs that are not sold over-the-counter. Aside from the question of the power and prestige of the doctors is the very alarming fact that most doctors have neither the training nor knowledge of drugs that the pharmacists do. This is amply documented in the book just referred to above. Many doctors get their drug education not by study but from the information supplied by detail men (salesmen) of the drug companies and from glossy drug company magazines and advertisements.

Here are some excerpts from a full-page two-color advertisement for Desyrel, an antidepressant, in the magazine *Medical Aspects of Human Sexuality*:

COMFORTABLE

There is minimal anticholinergic activity, cardiotoxicity is rare in patients free of cardiac disease, and there is no amphetamine-like CNS stimulation to disrupt therapy. The major portion of the daily dose may be given in the evening to place any possible sedative effect where it will do the most good . . . at bedtime.

PRESCRIBE EFFECTIVENESS WITH COMFORT

Desyrel helps your patient evoke an emotional environment and state of mind more receptive to your counseling and treatment. Achieve the level of therapeutic effect you desire, but without the incidence of disruptive effects older agents have been known to produce.

It convinces even a skeptic like me. Or how about Tranxene in the same magazine?

BRIEF SUMMARY OF PRESCRIBING INFORMATION

INDICATIONS—For management of anxiety disorders or short-term relief of symptoms of anxiety; for symptomatic relief of acute alcohol withdrawal; for adjunctive therapy in partial seizures.

Anxiety or tension associated with stress of everyday life usually does not require treatment with an anxiolytic. Effectiveness in long-term management of anxiety (over 4 months) not assessed by systematic clinical studies. The physician should periodically reassess usefulness for each patient.

INTERACTIONS—Potentiation may occur with ethyl alcohol, hypnotics, barbiturates, narcotics, phenothiazines, MAO inhibitors, other antidepressants. In bioavailability studies with normal subjects, concurrent administration of antacids at therapeutic levels did not significantly influence bioavailability of TRANXENE.

TRUST TRANXENE

Get with it! Don't be a doubting Thomas! These advertisements sound so authoritative that many doctors accept them as gospel. But we must remember that when thalidomide was introduced in 1958 by a German firm it quickly won acceptance in Germany as one of the safest sedatives ever discovered. And even though its use was not authorized in the United States, some Americans smuggled it in. In 1959, 12 children were born with seal-like flippers instead of arms and legs. There were 83 such cases in 1960 and 302 in 1961. At least 50% of the mothers of these children had used thalidomide during their pregnancies.

All drugs are potentially dangerous even if they have been adequately tested. This is true of over-the-counter drugs (OTC) as well as prescriptions. To advertise any drug in newspapers, magazines, radio, or television is in itself a pernicious practice because the message without sufficient caveats reaches children and others who may be incapable of exercising proper judgment.

One of the latest methods of promotion developed by drug companies is to print attractive brochures describing in glowing terms the efficacy of particular drugs and place them in physicians' offices so that patients can read them, be suitably impressed, and ask the doctors to prescribe them. This method of enlisting the physicians as part of the drug company's sales force is an invasion of the relationship between doctor and patient and should not be tolerated.

The reason for the large advertising expenditures is not difficult to discover. Drug companies constitute the most profitable manufacturing industry in the country, earning a higher rate of profit than the glamorous automobile, television, and computer companies. This has been documented in hearings before the Subcommittee on Antitrust and Monopoly of the Committee on the Judiciary, Eighty-Sixth Congress, 1960.

The following tabulation, based on figures extracted from *Hoover's Profiles of Over 500 Major Corporations,* 1991, indicates the relative profitability of two pharmaceutical companies and several other types of business enterprises:

| | Millions of Dollars | | |
Company	Sales	Profit	% Profit
Merck & Co., Inc. (world's leader in prescription drug sales)	$6,551	$2,236	34.1%
Pfizer, Inc. (5th in U.S. major drug sales)	$5,672	$952	16.8%
Ford Motor Co.	$96,146	$6,029	6.3%
General Motors Corp.	$124,993	$13,275	10.6%
General Electric Co.	$53,884	$7,036	13.1%

Most countries do not grant patent protection to companies manufacturing and distributing drugs. The United States is one of the few countries that does. Obviously this is of tremendous value to the drug companies granted such patents. And the irony of it is that most of the research and development expense of developing such drugs is shouldered by the United States government and not the drug companies. For example, as reported by *Medical World News* of June 18, 1965, by that year the government spent much more than $1,000,000,000 of the total of research costs of $1,700,000,000.

Another interesting fact reported by *Con$umer New$week* in October, 1972, is that two researchers from the Department of Health, Education and Welfare determined that drug companies in the United States sold drugs to foreign countries at prices far below the prices in the United States. Many drugs referred to here sold at 50% or less in foreign countries.

One of the most obvious and flagrant methods of gouging the public is to prescribe drugs by trade name rather than generic name, the latter being incredibly cheaper. The doctors go along with this practice because the drug industry rewards the AMA and the doctors by paying millions of dollars for advertisements in their medical journals.

In their book *Pills, Profits, and Politics*, University of California Press, 1974, Drs. Philip Lee and Milton Silverman discuss with devastating detail the failures of drug efficacy and drug quality. They also discuss the adverse reactions to drugs carelessly administered or administered without sufficient knowledge. In *The American Connection*, by John Pekkanen, Allyn and Bacon, Inc., 1973, the author refers to the relationship between the Pharmaceutical Manufacturers Association (PMA) and the AMA. He states, page 138:

Dr. John Adriani, an independent medical professor and anesthesiologist from New Orleans and former chairman of the AMA Council on Drugs, puts it bluntly: "The drug industry has the AMA in its hip pocket." The drug industry's demands are funnelled through the PMA, which deals with the AMA on a day-to-day basis. Their relationship is so tight on the policy-making level that since the PMA was founded in 1958, both its presidents have held prominent positions with the AMA before heading the PMA. It's the revolving door policy.

Since the early 1960s the drug industry had annually spent about $10 million a year on advertising in the AMA publications, including the lay magazine *Today's Health,* which means the drug industry supports about one-half of the AMA's annual budget.*

In the U.S. Senate, Special Committee on Aging, *Nursing Home Care in the United States: Failure in Public Policy,* 1975, it was reported that there is substantial phony billing or inflated charging for prescription drugs. In pharmaceutical service, these practices are often related to kickback arrangements.

Closely related to pharmaceutical charges are clinical laboratory charges. In this area, profiteering, fraud, and abuse are rampant. The following excerpts are taken from a report prepared by the Subcommittee on Aging, United States Senate, 1976.

EVIDENCE OF FRAUD AND ABUSE

In the past 2 years an increasing number of state officials have indicated concern about the potential for fraud and abuse among clinical labs participating in Medicaid. Major investigations have been conducted in New Jersey and New York. Providers have been accused of abusing the program in several other states including Michigan, California, and Pennsylvania. The Committee's investigation focused on Illinois.

A. TESTIMONY OF EDMOND L. MORGAN,
EXECUTIVE SECRETARY, ILLINOIS CLINICAL
LABORATORY ASSOCIATION

At the September 26, 1975 Subcommittee hearing, Mr. Morgan

* Pekkanen, John, *The American Connection.* Copyright © 1973 by Allyn and Beacon, Inc. Reprinted by permission.

testified that members of the Illinois Clinical Laboratory Association (ICLA) were "distressed" about the "practices of many unethical laboratory facilities which tend to question the integrity of all clinical laboratories in Illinois."

He said that kickbacks and other abuses were common nationwide, citing there has been a major fraud investigation underway in New York by the U. S. Attorney's office. He added:

"It has recently come to our attention that certain criminal elements are involved in the purchase of laboratories and also involved in establishing factoring agencies.

"Our Association estimates that approximately $10 to $12 million are annually being siphoned out of the health care dollar in Illinois through the padding of laboratory bills and overutilization.

"Of the $600 million annually spent in Illinois for health care through public aid for all services, it is estimated that approximately $100 to $125 million is being siphoned out through some form of fraud and unethical billing practices."

In addition, Mr. Morgan stated:

"Most of the Medicare and Medicaid patients for which laboratories perform services reside in nursing homes or convalescent and rest homes."

Mr. Morgan asserted that overutilization had become the rule rather than the exception in inner city facilities. He said that in such areas a pharmacy and a clinical lab will make joint arrangement with a clinic or medical doctors for a flow of tests. More often than not, according to Mr. Morgan, the physicians work for clinic owners. (There are a few requirements in any state with respect to ownership of a laboratory; most laws focus on the qualifications of the operator.) Clinic owners often hire physicians under contracts and "encourage" them to order unnecessary tests to generate income for a lab in which they might have an interest or in order to maximize the amount of the kickback they might receive from a laboratory (in exchange for sending them all the lab business of the clinic).

Morgan testified:

"In 1974 myself and my administrative assistant along with two special investigators assigned to the Legislative Advisory Commission to the Illinois Department of Public Aid inspected and investigated six laboratories chosen at random of whom we suspected of engaging in kickbacks and overutilization patterns in order to reap substantial sums of money."

1. Norven Medical Laboratory, a very small laboratory, was billing for numerous tests not performed in this facility. This laboratory was also billing for large sums of money without adequate facilities to perform these services.
2. D. J. Laboratory-Monticello Laboratory also was billing for substantial sums of money without adequate facilities or personnel.
3. Chicago Medical Laboratory, same pattern existed in this facility and had no proper directors or supervisors.
4. Division Medical Laboratory, also heavily involved in gross utilization with suspected kickbacks to physician clients.

The same publication describes and details similar conversations. It also explains how other states display the same pattern.

Hospitals frequently buy drugs at a discount but seldom pass the savings on to the patients, thus giving a greater profit to the hospitals, even though most of them are tax-exempt.

At the beginning of 1984 I discussed these examples of fraud and abuse, as well as those described in other chapters, with William Halamandaris, one of the investigators for the subcommittee. I asked him whether these abuses had been curbed as the result of the hearings. "On the contrary," he replied, "they have gotten worse."

Once more we can see the drug companies, clinical laboratories, physicians, nursing homes, and hospitals overcharging patients and insurance payers, both government and other, while the taxpayers foot the bill and the governmental agencies neglect enforcement. Meanwhile, politicians and the news media in many cases claim that aid to the indigent is bankrupting the country and should be drastically curtailed.

The *Wall Street Journal* of May 25, 1984, reports "Prices of Prescription Drugs Soar After Years of Moderate Increases." I can understand the first five words of the title of the article, but I do not comprehend the last five words. However, the article reports that since 1980 drug prices rose overall by 37%, whereas prices of all other commodities rose by 13%.

An official of the government's Health Care Financing Administration, which is in charge of Medicare and Medicaid payments for drugs, is quoted in the same article as saying that drug costs have been rising faster than other medical costs.

Per the Bureau of Labor Statistics, in 1983, the price of cancer therapy drugs rose 24%, sedatives 21.7%, and cardiovascular medicines 12.5%. And no one, in the industry or out of it, claims that this is justified by increased costs. Apparently it is a matter of what in the old days was called "profiteering." I can't think of a more accurate name for what is happening in the drug industry today.

And what is the government doing about it? *Lamenting.*

Health Care Insurance Fraud and Abuse

Insurance is probably one of the most secure businesses in the world. It is a device to handle risk. Its purpose is to replace uncertainty with certainty by promising to reimburse the insured in the event that certain occurrences result in losses during a specific time period. Because the insurance companies rely on large samplings, it is possible for them to make very accurate estimates of the normal frequency of the events involved. As a result they can set insurance rates very realistically so that their income can be sufficient to meet the liabilities when they occur and to secure a very handsome profit in addition.

Life insurance, fire insurance, and various types of business insurance have been with us in this country for a long time. Health insurance, however, is relatively new and is expanding rapidly. There are various methods of providing health insurance. The following quotation from "Insurance" in the *Encyclopaedia Britannica,* lists some of the variations*:

Private health insurance—In many countries health insurance has become a governmental institution. In some, doctors are employed, directly or indirectly, by a government agency on a full-time or part-time salaried basis, and health facilities are owned or operated by the government. This is the practice in Australia, Brazil, Canada, Chile, Greece, Ireland, Mexico, New Zealand, Sweden, Turkey, and the former Communist countries

* From "Insurance" in *Encyclopedia Britannica,* 15th edition (1974), 9:652. Reprinted by permission.

of Europe. In other countries the government pays for medical care provided by private physicians; these countries include Austria, Denmark, West Germany, The Netherlands, Norway, and Spain. In some countries private health insurance programs exist along with, or as part of, the government program. Various combinations of programs are possible, and it is difficult to summarize all the arrangements. The United States provides government-run medical services in veterans' hospitals and mental hospitals; it also has a governmental health insurance program under the Social Security Act amendments of 1965; but most health insurance in the United States still consists of private programs. Much private health insurance in the U. S. is operated on a group basis, generally through groups of employees whose payments may be subsidized by their employer.

In the United States, health care is not a right. If it were, people would get the health care they need without recourse to private insurance companies. However, the debate of health care as a right versus health care as a privilege is not the issue at hand—it is health care insurance fraud and abuse. The same *Encyclopaedia Britannica* article referred to above describes some of the problems encountered when dealing with private health care insurance contracts, and I shall mention a few:

* They are quite restricted in coverage, to the point that many consider them inadequate for modern times.
* They lend themselves to abuses such as overutilization of coverage, multiple policies, and insuring for more than 100% of expected loss.
* They help to escalate rising medical costs by encouraging physicians to charge more for insured procedures because of the certainty of payments.

Blue Cross and Blue Shield in 1986 had combined national net revenue of $43.5 billion. How did it happen that Blue Cross, which first saw the light of day in 1929, and Blue Shield, which under the name of California Physicians Service, was organized in 1939, experienced such an unprecedented growth in a relatively short span of time? That can be understood only if we look briefly at the history of the health care industry of this country. We shall do so even though some of this has been covered previously. From 1875 to 1915,

American medical institutions had a phenomenal growth, and by 1920 the pattern of our hospital system had crystallized, but by 1931, after the Depression, according to AMA data, only 62% of the beds in voluntary hospitals were occupied.[6] The AHA solved the problem to some extent by creating the Blue Cross, which was a logical extension of the small voluntary plans for the prepayment of medical expenses. Of the 39 Blue Cross plans established in the early 1930s, 22 were completely financed by hospitals and five were partially financed by them.

For reasons that have never been explained or justified, Blue Cross has been exempt from federal taxation under Section 501(c)(4) of the Internal Revenue Code, which provides that "civic leagues or organizations not organized for profit but operated exclusively for the promotion of social welfare" shall be exempt. As Blue Cross is an insurance company in direct competition with profit-making commercial companies that are not exempt, the ruling seems curious. The social welfare referred to appears to be the social welfare of the hospitals and doctors running them and benefitting financially thereby. Blue Cross has also been found to be exempt from tax by the various states in which the entities operate. The same thing is true of Blue Shield, which will be discussed later.

Blue Cross plans differed from other commercial plans by paying hospitals directly, which was a financial bonanza to the hospitals. Other plans paid the patients, some of whom never got around to paying the hospitals. Obviously the hospitals preferred Blue Cross. With the advent of Medicare and Medicaid, the function of Blue Cross became vastly more important than it had been. With a little bit of help from its friends, AHA and the American Medical Association (AMA), Blue Cross became the fiscal intermediary for the federal and state governments to pay claims by hospitals for Medicare and Medicaid services to patients. Blue Shield succeeded in getting the same assignment for services by doctors. The logical question at this point is why do the governmental agencies need fiscal intermediaries? They do not require such intermediaries for defense expenditures or for other purchases. The answer is simple if not pretty. The AMA and the AHA, with their powerful lobbies, want, insist on and get their bills paid with a minimum of trouble, examination, and delay. They are so powerful that for them it is the best of all possible worlds.

There is practically no federal or state supervision or examination of what the two Blues spend in performing these functions. For example, in New York, the superintendent of insurance of that state had conducted an audit of Blue Cross in the 1960s. The court criticized the superintendent as follows:

> [There is no reason for his] assuming the role of a mere automaton, blindly approving mathematically correct adjustments (i.e., rate increases) in the formula. . . . The Superintendent does not and will not examine into the reasonableness and propriety of payments made to member hospitals by [Blue Cross]. Taking refuge behind the strict letter of the law, he asserts that it is his duty to determine the reasonableness of "rates" of payments, not reasonableness of payments themselves. He argues that examining into actual payments would be an overwhelming task.

After consideration of New York's reasonable cost reimbursement formula for hospitals, the court continued:

> Overseeing and controlling this mathematical labyrinth is [Blue Cross]. . . . So complete and unfettered is this control that when [Blue Cross] discovered that substantial overpayments had mistakenly been made to member hospitals, its review committee decided that no repayment was necessary but that these amounts would be set off against supplemental payments that might come due to the hospitals in succeeding years.

> The Superintendent, meanwhile, would have us believe that he is to play absolutely no part in supervising or controlling this plan. He would have us believe that it is none of his concern whether payments are based on mistaken facts, fictitious charges, fictitious employees or even fictitious patients; nor that he should be concerned with making any independent evaluation of the reasonableness of . . . any of the myriad other details which would require him to go beyond the four corners of the balance sheet and ledger book. . . .

> Both [Blue Cross] and the Superintendent seem intent on adopting the notion that no matter how costly operations become, for whatever reasons, eventually and inevitably, [Blue Cross] subscribers will shoulder the load. Small wonder that subscriber rates have increased 124% in the past five years.

That was New York in the 1960s. How about California at the present time? When I visited the Supervisory Insurance Examiner of the Department of Insurance of the State of California, I asked him if the department audits Blue Cross, Blue Shield, and the other health insurance companies. I was told that they do perform such audits on a biannual basis but that the results are not open to the public because they are considered to be confidential. When I questioned this he replied that in the future they would be open to the public, but that would be several years from now. However, as a special dispensation he did allow me to look at the 1983 audit briefly. The short examination was not sufficient for me to draw any conclusions. From what he said, though, I gathered that further examination would have been useless.

He explained that their audits were intended to accomplish two things:

1. Is the insurance company solvent? If not, the Department may recommend steps to help attain solvency.
2. Do the figures on the books agree with the figures of their statements?

From an auditing point of view these are strange objectives. In response to my query as to whether the department took action on excessive costs that would result in higher premium and possibly insolvency problems, the answer was no! Apparently the only action by the department in the case of possible insolvency would be to recommend higher premiums for the consumers.

Because the department does not do anything about the financial statements in any case, why bother to match book and record costs?

I was curious about how the department controlled insurance premium rates. I was told that generally the law of supply and demand or the market demand took care of that. However, if the rate increase was to be greater than 25%, that required a review by the department. It is obvious how that hurdle can be cleared; increase rates by 24%.

Next I inquired who runs Blue Cross. Who are the members of the Board of Directors? The Examiner quoted Section 11498(a) of the California Insurance Code, which states:

Not more than one-third of the directors of such a corporation shall be duly appointed representatives of hospitals with which the corporation has contracts for the rendering of hospital services and duly qualified and licensed practicing physicians holding valid and unrevoked certificates to practice medicine and surgery or physician and surgeon certificates, issued under the provisions of the State Medical Practice Act in the State of California. Not less than two-thirds of the directors of such a corporation shall be duly appointed representatives of the public.

I looked at the list for 1983. In addition to executives of hospitals there were doctors, lawyers, bank executives, business executives, and one trade union executive.

Apparently there were no women. The closest thing to a normal working man was the trade union executive. When I questioned the composition of the board I was told that these executives were experienced people who really knew what the public needed.

This was California. How about other areas in the country? In Philadelphia in the early 1980s, the 32 members of the Board of Directors of Blue Cross were:

Directors of banking and finance	12
Major real estate company executives	2
President of hospital supply company	1
Organized labor executives	2
Other business executives	15
TOTAL	32

The pattern is the same throughout the country. Typical board members are white, male, over 40, and wealthy.

As has been mentioned earlier, Blue Cross and Blue Shield administered most of the Medicare and Medicaid programs. What did they charge for this service as fiscal intermediaries of the federal and state governmental agencies? No one really knows. No federal standards were set up. What emerges is a chaotic picture of different rates in different states. There has been little or no federal supervision or audits. No one knows how well the various programs work. To illustrate this here is an excerpt from a book, *Blue Cross—What Went Wrong?*, published by the New Haven and London, Yale University Press in 1974:

Apart from these weaknesses in the system, there are problems that arise directly from the use of local Blue Cross plans in Medicaid administration, the most common being unaccountable and excessive payments to them. An HEW Audit Agency study describes, as "one illustrative example," the contract between the Texas State Department of Public Welfare (TSDPW) and Group Health Services (GHS), Inc., a subsidiary of Blue Cross/Blue Shield of Texas.

The only information provided TSDPW as the basis for determining GHS administrative costs was a one page summary of estimated costs which totaled over $3 million. The summary listed 10 administrative costs items, one of which was "provider audits" at an estimated cost of $225,000. As of the date of our audit, no provider audits had been made and there were no firm plans to make any. . . .

Another item was $1.2 million for "data processing." . . . There was no documentation available to show the relationship between estimated costs expected under the terms of the contract and the $1.2 million.

Another item in the amount of $260,000 was listed for "executive, administrative, and legal" costs, but no itemization or allocation was ever requested or provided to show whether this amount was reasonably spent and reasonably attributable to the Medicaid operation.

Another HEW Audit Agency study found that there was no way of knowing whether the administrative costs paid to Delaware Blue Cross were reasonable or properly charged to Medicaid. The contract required Blue Cross to submit biannual reports showing costs and expenses together with supporting data, but Blue Cross failed to submit the information. The state agency accepted the Blue Cross figures without question, because it did not have the personnel to determine their accuracy. The state auditor of accounts audited the Blue Cross books but did not attempt to check the accuracy of its apportionments.*

I do not wish to create the impression that Blue Cross and Blue Shield are the only insurance companies taking advantage of a public frightened by the prospect of bankruptcy; the number of such companies is legion. In 1981 the federal government issued a report on *Cancer Insurance: Exploiting Fear for Profit* (an examination of dread disease insurance). Some of their conclusions (I am listing only 6 of 33) are as follows:[7]

1. A disproportionate number of cancer insurance policies are sold to the elderly.
2. Some companies improperly imply an endorsement for their product from the American Cancer Society.
3. Insurance companies that sell cancer insurance use fear tactics to induce people to buy policies.

*Sylvia A. Law, Blue Cross: What Went Wrong?, 2nd ed. (New Haven & London: Yale University Press, 1976). Reprinted by permission.

4. Some companies exaggerate statistics to promote cancer insurance sales.
5. Some companies selling cancer insurance belabor cancer costs.
6. Some companies selling cancer insurance belittle basic health insurance coverage.

One of the most important conclusions is the following:

As a result of this investigation, the Committee concluded that the critics of cancer insurance were justified in their complaints. It is apparent that cancer and other dread disease policies have very limited economic value and that there are significant abuses associated with the marketing of these forms. There is good reason to question the sale of these policies to senior citizens in particular and the Congress or the States may wish to prohibit the practice.

The report then proceeds to list about 100 insurance companies who solicit specified/dread disease policies (1978). And the report then calculates that an average policy cost of $75 per year, the total cancer insurance market in 1981 may have amounted to $3 billion a year in sales, or more than 6% of total American health care expenditures. *Although more can be said on insurance company fraud and abuse, I believe we can conclude with that example of $3 billion waste.*

Physicians' Fraud and Abuse

Once again I wish to stress the fact that most physicians adhere to ethical standards; unfortunately the number who do not is far from negligible. I also wish to distinguish between two types—sins of omission and sins of commission. A suitable illustration is the song that Eliza Dolittle sings to Henry Higgins in *My Fair Lady:*

> You'll be swimming in the sea
> And you get a cramp a little way from me.
> When you yell you're going to drown
> I'll get dressed and go to town!

What do we have here? A sin of commission or a sin of omission? In this case, it is not an example of "either," "or." It is an example of *both*. Because of the doctor's exclusive right in our society to admit or not admit a patient to a hospital, he may and sometimes does condemn patients to death, as we have seen in the Hill-Burton cases discussed earlier in this book. His exclusive right to prescribe drugs, to perform procedures that can be performed as well and far cheaper by well-trained paramedical personnel contributes to the unnecessary inflation of medical costs. The refusal of most doctors to accept the possibility of reforming our shameful health care system or consider replacing it with a better one is a demonstration of myopia at best and greed at worst. The result is clearly, and it should be stated clearly, that our present health care system benefits the medical profession financially, even though it impairs professional integrity, deprives a large segment of proper medical care, and in many cases the avoidance of suffering and premature death, while at the same time defeating cost containment.

That is a strong indictment, it is true, but now let us look at *A Public Citizen Health Research Group Report, June 1990,* by Nicole Simmons, Phyllis McCarthy, and Sidney Wolfe. It is entitled *6892 Questionable Doctors Disciplined by States or the Federal Government.*

In June 1990 there were 540,000 medical doctors in the United States; the 6,892 doctors disciplined constitute only 1.3%. That, however, is not the whole story. For example, Harvard researchers studied New York state hospitals in 1984, and found a number of patients were injured, and some died because of medical negligence.[8] Translating that to the nation as a whole we are talking about 234,000 injuries and 80,000 deaths. Other studies tend to confirm these findings, indicating that the 6,892 questionable doctors are only the tip of the iceberg. The doctors were disciplined for overprescribing or misprescribing drugs, criminal convictions, alcohol or drug abuse, sexual abuse of a patient, or sexual misconduct. Since many abuses of this type are never reported, or disciplinary action is slow, and at times never takes place, we can safely assume that the number of actual cases of negligence, fraud, and abuse are much more frequent than reported here. And when all of these result in death, injury, or lack of proper medical care, the expenditures result in substantial waste.

And Where Are the Watchdogs?

They are supposed to be protecting the public. Lawyers should be interpreting the law so that the public gets what the law says it is entitled to, but the lawyers are too busy protecting the health care providers. The certified public accountants should be presenting figures and statements that show whether or not the public is getting the health care to which it is entitled, and whether the health care providers are fulfilling their contractual obligations, but we have seen that in the Hill-Burton cases, they were more concerned with protecting their clients. Recent events in the savings and loan debacle prove decisively that CPAs can be led astray because of their loyalty to their clients. A shocking example of CPA irresponsibility can be found in the case of the San Francisco investment bank Hambrecht & Quist, its chairman, former chairman, and the accounting firm Coopers & Lybrand, one of the largest CPA firms in the country. A Texas jury found them guilty of fraud and negligence and ordered the defendants to pay $29 million in actual damages and $530 million in punitive damages. Coopers & Lybrand were found liable for $200 million in punitive damages (*San Francisco Chronicle*, February 5, 1992, pp. B1 and B2). The plaintiffs were 100 investors. One more time it raises the question, "Whose interest are the CPAs protecting—their clients' or the public's?

The various governmental agencies spend most of their time drafting confusing laws and regulations, conducting surveys, decrying abuses, making recommendations, and promising to contain costs and insure the uninsured. Regulation of fraud and abuse, they say, and repeat, and repeat, will follow the next survey.

Where are the watchdogs? They are there all right, but they are watching the wrong way.

9. Preventive Medicine

"Preventive medicine" as used here is not the same thing as the "prevention of disease." The latter term embraces such measures as the elimination of pollution, governmental supervision of health providers, etc. What I mean by preventive medicine is the specific medical procedures health care providers should develop to prevent disease. The procedures on which I shall concentrate in this chapter are prenatal examinations and treatments; abortion; treatment of tobacco, alcohol and drug abuse; health education in schools and throughout life; disease and drug research; lead poisoning; and AIDS.

We are all familiar with the maxim that "an ounce of prevention is worth a pound of cure." Unfortunately, it is seldom true; it may be worth nothing if it is insufficient or not properly enforced. In 1711, in *An Essay on Man,* Alexander Pope said:

> A little learning is a dangerous thing; drink deep or taste not the Pierian spring. [Pieria was a center of learning in Macedonia, Greece.]

And Robert Browning in a poem, "By the Fireside," in 1855, wrote:

> Oh, the little more and how much it is!
> And the little less, and what worlds away!

From my point of view, they were both correct.

Prenatal Examinations and Treatments

In 1987, according to the World Health Organization (WHO), approximately 500,000 women die each year of pregnancy-related causes, more than 98% occurring in the so-called developing world.[1] Actually this is a sad misnomer. The so-called developing world is more accurately described as the "undeveloped world," because most of the nations are *not* developing. A few may be developing, but the rest are remaining stationary or are defunct or dying. As reported by Allan Rosenfield, M.D., Dean, School of Public Health, DeLamar Professor of Public Health, Columbia University, the five major causes of maternal deaths in those countries are obstructed labor, postpartum hemorrhage, pregnancy-induced hypertension, postpartum sepsis, and illegal botched abortions. Much of this problem arises because there are too few doctors, trained paramedical personnel, efficient hospitals, and legal abortions, even in the urban areas.[2] In the rural areas, there are practically no medical facilities, and, in many cases, pregnant women about to give birth cannot get to an urban hospital in time; many deliver babies without any prenatal care or even without a traditional birth attendant or relative in attendance. Dr. Rosenfield concludes that we can change the picture for the better in the undeveloped countries by utilizing aseptic techniques, providing more health education in the communities, establishing maternity waiting homes so women at risk can stay near a hospital during the last weeks of pregnancy, performing operations to correct pelvic abnormalities where needed, providing a network of facilities to take care of blood transfusions, cesarean sections, antibiotics, and above all: prenatal care, abortions where needed, and a budget adequate to handle all this.[3] This is not revolutionary; it is, or should be, normal good medical practice.

The U.S. record is much better, of course. According to the U.S. health statistics, the maternal deaths in childbirth in 1987 amounted to 6.6 per 1,000.[4] This compares to 100 to 200 deaths per 1,000 in the undeveloped countries. However, a closer look at the U.S. figures is very informative. At this point, I will present both infant and maternal mortality rates in the U.S. in 1987:

	Deaths per 1,000 Live Births	
	Infant	**Maternal**
Total per 1,000 live births	10.1	6.6
Total white	8.6	5.1
Total black and other	15.9	12.0
Total black	17.9	14.2

The variations in the tabulation make it abundantly clear that what is needed in the United States in ghetto areas and depressed rural areas is the same infusion of facilities and personnel as in the undeveloped countries. As John Donne said in *Devotions Upon Emergent Occasions* (1624):

> Therefore never send to know for whom
> the bell tolls; it tolls for thee.

And how does the government plan to fight infant mortality? According to the *New York Times,* Louis Sullivan, Secretary of Health and Human Services, said the administration plans to take $24 million from community health centers and $34 million from the existing maternal and child health service block grants this year to implement President Bush's proposal to combat infant mortality.[5] I believe this plumbs the depths of inanity! There are several other equally ridiculous plans.

Abortions as Preventive Medicine

Legal abortions in the U.S. are necessary for a number of reasons:

* Amniocentesis may indicate the undesired birth of a defective infant.
* Giving birth to a child may in some cases endanger the life of a pregnant woman.
* A woman has the right to decide whether she wishes to have a child.
* It can prevent teenage girls from having unintended, unwanted infants, which in most cases places a heavy burden on society.
* The prevention of legal abortions, as the history in practically every country in the world indicates, leads to illegal abortions, many of which result in maternal fatalities.
* Women who test HIV positive run the risk of having a child infected with HIV.

Given this as a background, what should the medical profession be doing about it? Hippocrates, the so-called father of medicine (460–377 B.C.), provided the answer in no uncertain terms, and doctors observe the Hippocratic oath, which states that the physician's primary ethical and professional duty is to place the interest of his patient first—not the dictates of the Catholic church or any other church. In this case it means that the physician should perform abortions needed to protect the physical and psychological health and the civil rights of his patients. He should oppose restrictive legislation.

We should also emphasize the fact that abortions must be kept legal as an alternative since other methods of birth control may fail or are not available. In the United States, the medical establishment has been lax in researching new, cheap, effective methods of birth control. If they did so, the necessity for abortions would be greatly diminished.

Very recently a new pill, RU-486, was developed.[6] It is not an abortion pill but an unpregnancy pill. It breaks down the embryo's bond to the uterine wall and the embryo is washed from the body. It can prevent pregnancy without surgical abortion, which, under sanitary conditions, is quite safe. However, in many undeveloped countries and in the back streets of U.S. cities where abortion is banned, the risk is great, and well over 50 million abortions are performed annually worldwide, half of them illegally.

RU-486 is useful in cases where contraception has not been used or has failed, and the pregnancy is not wanted. *RU-486 is legal in France, Britain, and China, but not in the United States.*

Treatment of Tobacco, Alcohol and Drug Abuse

There is no better way to introduce the subject of tobacco abuse than to quote a passage from a U.S. governmental source:[7]

Smoking and Health

Cigarette smoking is the largest single preventable cause of illness and premature death in the United States. Cigarette smokers have a 70 percent higher overall death rate than non-smokers, and tobacco is associated with an estimate in excess of 300,000 premature deaths per year. The major single cause of cancer mortality in the United States is cigarette smoking, contributing to more than 100,000 cancer deaths annually. Smoking is a causal factor in coronary heart disease and arteriosclerotic peripheral vascular disease and is also the most important cause of chronic obstructive lung disease. Cigarette smoking acts synergistically with alcohol to increase the likelihood of cancer of the larynx, esophagus, and oral cavity, with other coronary risk factors such as hypercholesteremia to aggravate cardiovascular risk, and with oral contraceptives to increase the risk of coronary heart disease and some forms of cerebrovascular disease. During pregnancy, cigarette smoking can increase the risk of spontaneous abortion, retarded fetal growth, and even fetal or neonatal death.

That is a comprehensive condemnation of the use of tobacco made in 1983. The two most important types of tobacco are flue-cured, types 11–14 and burley, type 31. According to the annual monthly reports of the Internal Revenue Service, U.S. Department of Agriculture, and the Commerce Department, reported in 1983, the United States price-support operations in 1981 amounted to $1.64 per pound for tobacco producers. And why? The following quotation is taken from an analysis by the U.S. Department of Agriculture:

Tobacco has been important to the American economy since the 17th-century settlement of the English colonies in Virginia. Today it is the sixth most valuable agricultural crop harvested in the United States and a mainstay in the agricultural economies of at least seven states.

Tobacco growing has prospered in recent years; in 1978, farmers produced a near-record tonnage and received the highest prices in history. The total value of the crop was $2.7 billion; of this, approximately half will be used in the manufacture of American cigarettes, and the rest is destined for export to American and other companies manufacturing tobacco products abroad.

The same type of claim could be made about slavery in the United States.

Two significant statements are relevant here:

1. The government, by sins of commission and omission, increases the development of cancer in the United States.
2. Our health system is firmly committed to a policy of attempting to cure disease and not prevent it. The same policy is true, incidentally, in our income tax laws. A medical expense is deductible if incurred to attempt to cure and not prevent. One of my clients who wished to quit smoking asked me if the cost of a cruise to Alaska on a vessel with no cigarettes aboard was a deductible medical expense. The answer was no. The IRS definitely says so. My advice

was, "Increase your smoking. After you develop cancer, or emphysema if you are lucky, your medical expenses, probably ineffective, will be deductible."

One of the more egregious contradictions here is that the public makes contributions to the Cancer Fund and the various branches of our government, and hospitals waste a lot of money trying to stem the ravages of smoking, which is supported in part by the federal government. And the game goes on. As reported in *The San Francisco Chronicle,* March 12, 1991, p. A 9, tobacco industry contributions and lobbying increased more than eightfold from $563,983 in 1986 to $3.9 million in 1991. What we are looking at is the waste of money by our government to support an industry that is poisoning the public, including teenagers. And there is the additional waste of treating the victims by hospitals, doctors, etc.

When Oedipus killed his father and then married his mother, there were extenuating circumstances; after all, consciously at any rate, Oedipus did not know that Laius was his father and Jocasta was his mother, nor did they know that Oedipus was their son. The actors in the tobacco tragedy know each other very well; there are no extenuating circumstances.

As we have noted, cigarette smoking is the major single cause of cancer mortality in the United States. According to the publication *Health, United States 1990,* issued by U.S. Department of Health and Human Services, Table 30, p. 92, selected death rates for malignant neoplasms (cancers) of the respiratory system were as follows:[8]

	Deaths per 100,000 Resident Population		
	1970	**1980**	**1988**
All ages	28.4	36.4	39.9
15–24 years	0.2	0.1	0.1
25–34 "	1.0	0.8	0.7
35–44 "	11.6	9.6	7.6
45–54 "	46.2	56.5	50.0
55–64 "	116.2	144.3	162.2
65–74 "	174.6	243.1	280.0
75–84 "	175.1	251.4	324.2

Although a few of the age brackets show some minor improvement, the general trend is a worsening of the problem.

Before proceeding, I wish to make it clear that the prevention of tobacco, alcohol, and drug abuse is not a question of the prohibition of the production or use of those substances. As we learned in this country, when the Volstead Act was passed in 1919, establishing the Prohibition Era (1919–1933), the prohibition was a complete failure.[9] The refusal of most citizens to obey the law led to the condoning of lawlessness, invasion of personal rights by federal agents, corruption of government officials, powerlessness of the courts, and a rash of crime and immense bootlegging profits. *It did not diminish the drinking of alcoholic beverages.* The preventive control of substance abuse requires education, not prohibition.

In 1956, the AMA stated that alcoholism was a disease, and in 1960 Dr. E. M. Jellinek wrote of the etiology of "alcoholism" as a disease; it has been named by some as Jellinek's disease, although there is still no consensus in the medical profession that it is a disease.[10] Those who refer to it as such feel that the term converts what many regard as a sin into a physical problem. But sin or disease, it is indeed a very serious problem.

The Diagnostic and Statistical Manual of Mental Disorders, DSM-III[11] asserts that the following organic mental disorders are attributed to the ingestion of alcohol: alcohol intoxication, alcohol idiosyncratic intoxication, alcohol withdrawal, alcohol withdrawal delirium, alcohol hallucinosis, alcohol mental disorder, and dementia associated with alcoholism. As mentioned previously, the DSM manual is utilized to identify psychiatric problems by description and code number for diagnostic and insurance reimbursement reasons. The numbers associated with the mental disorders just listed are not relevant here. According to the same manual, alcohol intoxication accounts for at least one-half of all highway fatalities, numerous falls, household and industrial accidents, and the commission of criminal acts.[12] More than one-half of all murderers and their victims are believed to be intoxicated at the time of the act. It accounts for about one-fourth of all suicides, and the results of falls and accidents include fractures, subdural hematomas, and other types of brain trauma. Exposure to extreme weather leads to frostbite or sunburn and can suppress immune mechanisms, thus predisposing people to infections. One of the most important characteristics of alcohol dependence and concomitant abuse is that it usually occurs within the first five years of regular drinking, and that heavy drinking in adolescents is particularly likely to lead to later problems.

Now that we have described the immensity of the problem, it is time to find out what is being done to deal with it. The most visible organization is Alcoholics Anonymous (AA), which was founded in 1935 in Akron, Ohio. It has now spread to over 100 other countries. As it developed, a program of recovery from alcoholism was developed with 12 steps; the first step was the admission of powerlessness when confronted with alcohol. Most of the rest of the program called God or any higher power to help the alcoholic quit the drinking compulsion. Several facts stand out like neon lights: AA is not preventive medicine; it is basically religious rather than scientific. It is not a cure, but the development of avoidance techniques that may or may not be permanent.

Television, viewed by children, teenagers, and adults, constantly shows glamorous, sexually exciting young men and women drinking beer ecstatically; advertisements in glossy magazines, on billboards and in newspapers extol the virtues of expensive, high-proof alcoholic beverages being quaffed as an accompaniment to seduction or rape, depending on what kind of lawyer you have. And what is the medical profession doing to prevent this headlong drive in the direction of alcohol abuse? Practically nothing. The only word of advice can be found near the cash registers of liquor stores, bars, and super-markets:

Warning:
Drinking distilled spirits, beer, coolers, wine, and other alcoholic beverages may increase cancer risk and, during pregnancy, can cause birth defects.

Whoever is responsible for this warning, whether the medical profession or some branch of our government, is pretty casual about the whole thing, like, "Drink it, even if it's a cancer risk. We simply thought you might want to know." What the medical profession should be doing is mounting an intensive educational campaign in schools, in churches, in clubs, in the media, etc., to explain in imaginative, graphic detail with words, films, lectures, and anything else available, what the dangers are. They should also mount a campaign, or stimulate one, by governmental agencies to eliminate seductive programs and advertisements that encourage the consumption of alcoholic beverages. The fact that taxes on the manufacture and sale may be attractive to governmental branches because the taxes increase revenue should not be allowed to countenance the traffic in death, to say nothing of the taxpayers' money needed to pay for avoidable costs of all types.

Alcohol abuse and dependence are more common among members of the same family than in the general population, and evidence of a genetic factor is a more frequent occurrence of alcohol dependence in the young adopted children of parents with the disorder. As quoted in the book *Alcoholism, the Genetic Inheritance,* there are 17 million people in the U.S. suffering from alcoholism,[13] including 4.4 million children 13 to 17 years of age. In a school of 450 children, 100 have an alcoholic parent. The significance of these statistics is that if the medical profession should conduct an intensive research program to establish the genetic and social criteria for identifying those individuals at risk of alcoholism, it would be very helpful. After all, most people who drink alcoholic beverages do so socially and are not at risk. We should concentrate our use of preventive medicine to help those who *are* at risk. Saturation bombing is not necessary and would be wasteful.

Before proceeding, one additional problem should be addressed. Some physicians have a tendency to avoid meaningful discussions of alcoholic beverage consumption with their middle-income patients. If they discuss it at all, their questions are perfunctory, confined to, "How many drinks do you have a day? One? Two?" And that's that. A more serious approach might disclose a more serious problem.

Drug Abuse

Drugs, which are chemical substances that affect the functions of living things (I am not including alcohol, which we have already considered) are used in treating, preventing and diagnosing diseases. In the mid-19th century, a German pharmacologist, Oswald Schmiedeberg, known as the father of pharmacology, began the synthesis of drugs, and since that time we have seen many thousands of synthesized drugs.[14] In addition, we have many drugs of natural origin extracted from plants, animals, minerals, bacteria, and fungi. Many of them have been useful in treating diseases, alleviating physical and mental afflictions, and enhancing the enjoyment of life without deleterious results. However, when a person uses a drug uncontrollably for pleasure without regard to medicinal use and becomes addicted to it, we call that drug abuse. It is characterized by a pattern of pathological use, impairment in social or occupational functioning caused by the pattern of pathological use, and a duration, not necessarily continuous, of at least one month.[15]

In addition to substance abuse as one large category, we also have substance dependence, which is more severe than abuse, involving tolerance (increased amounts required) and withdrawal disorders. Aside from alcohol and tobacco, the drugs include barbiturates or similarly acting sedatives or hypnotics, opium derivatives, amphetamines, cannabis, cocaine, crack, phenocyclidine (PCP), hallucinogens, and similar products. It can also include such bizarre activities as glue-sniffing, benzene-sniffing, and excessive use of codeine, etc.

The drug currently blighting the United States is crack, a product easily produced from cocaine powder. Begun in the early '80s, crack has spread rapidly because it is relatively inexpensive as compared to cocaine. Cocaine powder required an investment of $75 per gram, whereas a hit of crack costs only $5. The rush (onset of euphoria), in the case of crack, begins about eight seconds after the smoke is inhaled, and lasts for 10 to 12 minutes. There are several reasons for its popularity. There was a great demand for smokable cocaine, desperate teenagers and minority unemployed adults found the sale of crack financially rewarding, the product was cheap, and the preparation was simple. It was estimated by the National Cocaine Hotline that by 1986, one million Americans had tried crack.[16] Rival gangs were formed, and vicious gunfights and murders erupted in struggles to control the lucrative market. Although some of the leaders have been jailed, and others have been convicted but are now fugitives, the crack problems go on, and will, until more energetic measures are instituted to eliminate the underlying causes.

Although we may be unable to quantify the evil results of the drug abuse, we are all aware of them. Millions of our people, adults in all walks of life, students in colleges, high schools, grade schools, dropouts, poverty-stricken members of minority groups, misguided people seeking relief from pain, psychological problems, boredom or aging disabilities, suffer from drug abuse. Because in many cases the purchase, ownership, or sale of drugs is illegal, prices are astronomical. Addicts may steal to get enough money to satisfy their habit, they may become drug dealers themselves, form gangs to protect their territory, and commit crimes of all kinds, including murder. It is unsafe to walk the streets in many parts of the country, and there is ample reason to believe that our Drug Enforcement Agency is itself involved in drug trafficking. As reported in the *San Francisco Chronicle,* August 14, 1991, pp. A 8-10, a drug enforcement agent is under investigation for a variety of illegal activities that include arranging for a key player in Oliver North's Iran-Contra network to be secretly flown out of Costa Rica, where he faced trial on drug trafficking charges. He is also being charged with gaining financially from his illegal activities in the drug business.

The United States is well aware of the drug abuse problem.[17] The U.S. Department of Health and Human Services (DHHS) publishes monographs that describe in great detail the problems inherent in drug abuse. The monograph discussed here was prepared by the Office for Substance Abuse Prevention and is cosponsored by the American Academy of Child and Adolescent Psychiatry. Perhaps the clearest way to illustrate this type of publication is to show the Table of Contents of one of them:

CONTENTS

Page

I have no quarrel with the coverage here, but there is reason to be disturbed by the final two sentences of the book, and I quote:

> Countless thousands of children and adolescents who are at risk or showing the early features of a disturbance remain untreated and unrecognized. *Unless we can take this initiative,* they will continue to suffer both during their childhood, and in many instances, during the years to come. [Author's emphasis.]

A sensible medical prevention program would conclude: *Now that we have taken the initiative, many will no longer suffer during their childhood and in many instances, during the years to come.*

Lead Poisoning

Lead poisoning is a condition caused by absorption of lead from the digestive tract, lungs, or skin. It occurs among children who eat chips of lead-based paint in deteriorating buildings and among people who work in lead-using industries. Starting with mild diarrhea, anemia, and irritability, it can lead unnoticed to convulsions, and if untreated, to death. Lead pipes, gasoline emissions, and run-down areas with intensive lead pollutants also contribute to lead poisoning. It is true that most gasoline used in automobiles in the U.S. is now lead-free. Some children suffering from lead poisoning exhibit signs of intellectual impairment.

About 20 years ago, the U.S. Department of Commerce estimated that 600,000 children in the United States had dangerous levels of lead in their blood, and simple measures were proposed to stop the incidence of this peril.[18] The three primary proposals were to keep children out of areas that had been coated with lead paints, to remove such paint, or to cover it. In the 20 years that have elapsed, the U.S. Agency for Toxic Substances estimates that 17% of the nation's urban children—about 2.4 million—have levels of lead in their blood above the levels considered safe by the U.S. Center for Disease Control.[19] Now and then children and neighborhoods are tested to determine how widespread is the danger from lead-based paints and soil saturated with lead. Most of the children who contract lead poisoning are poor and live in these unhealthy neighborhoods.

This subject needs little elaboration. All the analyses, surveys, and promises come through loud and clear, but as Mark Twain said in 1908, in a letter to an unidentified person, "Thunder is good, thunder is impressive; but it is lightning that does the work." To alter slightly a very famous phrase, *"Let there be lightning!"*

AIDS

Most of what has to be done to prevent AIDS has been covered in Chapter 5, but because AIDS can endanger and destroy our entire health care system, together with our financial stability, we should again emphasize the most salient requirements of a preventive program; and it must be understood that adequate governmental funding is essential. Without it, all we will experience is colossal waste of the inadequate expenditures we are now having.

1. Explanation of the AIDS epidemic to reach all segments of our society, including the illiterate population.
2. Early detection and treatment, which can help prevent the spread of the disease.

3. Facilitation of the use of sterile needles for IV drug users.
4. Extension of treatment to cure or help drug addicts.
5. Explanation of safe sex to reach adults and children at home, in the media, in schools in understandable explicit language.
6. Expanded research of etiology of the disease and of drugs to treat it.
7. Reduction of cost of medicines to treat it.
8. Expanded home care programs and facilities to house and treat.
9. Recognition of and treatment of women who have contracted the disease, and children born by them.

The preventive measures listed would unquestionably be very costly, but not nearly as costly as what we are faced with because we are not instituting a sensible program. As it is now, we must bear the cost of treatment in overburdened hospitals of the men, women, and children afflicted with preventable cases of AIDS. The same thing is true in the case of drug addicts. We also neglect to conduct an educational program designed to reach all segments of our population, thus making it a probability that many will become drug addicts, contract AIDS and infect others.

What we have said about preventive medicine related to AIDS is equally true of all the other problems we have discussed in this chapter. Lack of effective preventive medicine results in colossal waste. In that cogent phrase coined by Robert Burton in *The Anatomy of Melancholy,* in the 17th century, we are being *penny wise, pound foolish.*

One of the most frustrating aspects of preventive medicine is that governmental publications and books and pamphlets written by experts dedicated to improving the situation are replete with helpful suggestions, but there is no machinery in place to make it work. *The machinery is the right kind of national health insurance.*

Conclusion:
The Single-Payer Approach to
National Health Insurance
by Thomas S. Bodenheimer, M.D.

The people of the United States need a single public system of national health insurance (NHI). Just as we all have a Social Security card, we should all have a health security card, entitling us to care at home, at the doctors' office, hospital, or group practice of our choice.

Under such a system, everyone would be provided comprehensive health coverage, including preventive care, physicians' services, lab, X-ray, prescription drugs, hospital care, mental health care, and long-term care with an emphasis upon care at home. If you are one of the 37 million people without health insurance, you would be automatically insured. Clauses that say, "Your insurance will not cover preexisting illnesses" would be prohibited. You could not be rejected as uninsurable, nor could you have your health insurance cancelled.

You would have free choice of physician and other medical providers. If you are in a health maintenance organization (HMO), you could continue in your plan, though HMOs would be required to be nonprofit. Your doctor and hospital would not be allowed to send you a bill.

Now, many employees are offered a limited choice of HMOs or other restricted plans. Under a national health insurance program, health insurance would no longer be linked to employment. Whether you are rich or poor, employed or unemployed, sick or healthy, young or old, you would have a health insurance card giving you access to health care.

Patients would never see a hospital or a medical bill. The 19-page itemized hospital bill separately listing each intravenous bottle, aspirin, and lab test would become an extinct species. Families would no longer spend their weekends unscrambling Grandpa's Medicare and supplemental insurance bills. Rather, a single health care trust fund set up in each state, under federal guidelines, would pay each hospital a lump sum budget negotiated yearly with the hospital. Physicians would be paid fees by the health care trust fund. This health care trust fund is generally called the single payer of health care.

How Is National Health Insurance Financed?

How, in our deficit-laden society, will we come up with the funds to initiate such a program? In 1991 the nation spent over $600 billion on personal health care services. At least 20% of this sum, $120 billion, goes for administration—paper pushing by hundreds of insurance companies, more paper pushing by hospitals who have to bill hundreds of insurance companies, and yet more paper pushing by doctors billing those same hundreds of companies.[1] The replacement, within each state, of multiple insurers by a single health care trust fund will save the nation about $67 billion each year—ample money to insure all of the 37 million uninsured Americans and to improve the coverage of the 56 million underinsured.[2]

Where, exactly, does the money come from? There are two parts to this question: (1) what is the ideal financing system for the long run? and (2) how do we make the transition from our present system of health care financing to the ideal system?

The Ideal System

The ideal system is fair and simple. Fair means that your health care would be financed by a progressive tax, that is, a tax in which higher-income people pay a greater percentage of their income than lower-income people. Currently, lower-income people pay a far higher percentage of their income for health care than the wealthy. Fair also means that everyone is obligated to pay (with the amount based on income and wealth) and that everyone receives the same benefits (based on need for health care).

Simple means that health care would be paid for by one tax rather than the multitude of payments currently faced. The tax would be earmarked for health care so that one could be sure that health taxes paid would be spent for health care rather than for military purposes, for savings and loan bailouts, or for politicians' travel expenses.

What is the fairest and simplest tax? Currently, the federal individual income tax. However, if this tax were used to finance health care, it would need to be reformed to make it more fair. Over the past 10 years the tax load for the wealthiest people has gone down while the tax load for lower- and middle-income people has gone up. Also, the federal income tax would have to be changed so that a portion of it is earmarked for health care.

Many people will say, "I don't want to pay more taxes." But remember: under a tax-financed health program, you would not be paying insurance premiums or doctor and pharmacy bills. For the average family, payments for health care would be less than they are now.

The Transition Program

It is impossible to jump abruptly from our current health financing system to a single progressive tax, so we must devise a transition financing program to get from here to there.

Currently, health care is financed in three major ways, each paying for about one-third of the nation's health expenditures: (1) payments from employers and employees for private health insurance premiums and for Medicare, (2) taxes, and (3) individual payments for health insurance premiums and out-of-pocket expenses.

Under the transition program, (1) payments from employers and employees would continue, but would all be directed to the single payer in each state, and would be made more progressive (lower rates for small businesses and for lower-paid employees). For example, rather than General Motors paying Blue Cross for its employees' health insurance, GM would pay those same funds to the single payer. (2) Current taxes that support Medicaid, portions of Medicare, and other governmental health programs would continue, and would go to the single payer in each state. (3) Individual payments would be greatly reduced, and new taxes would be levied to take their place. The amount of new taxes would not exceed the sum total of health care payments that individuals currently make. The taxes (which would make the wealthy pay a greater percentage of their income than lower- and middle-income people) would be far more fair than individual health payments (which force lower-income people to pay a greater percentage of their income for health care than the wealthy).

Let's look a bit more closely at how your health care will be financed. Suppose you work for United Airlines, which pays for most of your health insurance. Under the NHI transition financing program, United Airlines would continue to pay, but would pay the single payer in the state where you live rather than pay a private insurance company. If you get sick and lose your job, your health insurance would continue. When you retire, you would receive Medicare as now, but the large coinsurance and deductible payments that currently burden Medicare beneficiaries would be eliminated and covered by taxes.

Many taxes are levied by the federal government; yet the single-payer health funds are at the state level. Formulas would be set up to ensure that money collected by the federal government would be paid to the state single payers in an equitable way.

Who Administers National Health Insurance?

Each state would establish a single insurer (single payer) that is federally mandated but locally controlled. States could experiment with the structure of the single insurer; some may wish to place it within a government agency, some may prefer a board elected by the citizens, and yet others may choose a commission elected or appointed by provider and consumer interests within the state. Other states may create a public enterprise that combines elements of a private business and a government agency.

It is extremely important that health care money be earmarked for health care and be kept separate from general government revenues. Health care funds must be spared the annual budgetary fights that take place on Capitol Hill and in state legislatures. Adequate increases in health funding (based on such factors as aging of the population, epidemics, advances in medical technology, and inflation) must be mandated by law.

Are we talking about socialized medicine? No. Most hospitals would continue to be privately owned, and outpatient care would be delivered by the same pluralistic mix of private physicians, health maintenance organizations (HMOs), community clinics, and local governmental health facilities we have now. The single-payer approach to national health insurance meshes public insurance and private medicine.

Will Prevention Be Emphasized?

The most important aspects of prevention lie outside the health care arena: elimination of poverty, good education, healthy diets, exercise, a ban on all cigarette advertising, clean air and water, reduction of toxic wastes, etc. We have to realize that the NHI cannot do everything, and will not directly impact on these matters.

Another form of prevention does lie within the scope of national health insurance: prenatal and well-baby care, childhood immunizations, Pap smears, breast exams and mammograms, cholesterol and blood pressure screening. These services should be of the highest priority. A national health insurance program that covers these services will eliminate financial barriers to preventive care. But in addition, primary care must be adequately funded and reimbursed so that personnel are available to provide these preventive services. We do not want a health insurance program that overemphasizes high-tech specialty procedures at the expense of preventive care.

How Will High Quality Care Be Guaranteed?

Quality of care can be divided into (1) ensuring access to care, (2) eliminating inappropriate care, and (3) establishing procedures that help health care professionals continuously improve the care they provide.

(1) *Ensuring access to care.* A number of studies show that people without health insurance, or people with inadequate health insurance such as Medicaid, receive lower quality care than people who are adequately insured. The single-payer approach to national health insurance will provide everyone equally with adequate health insurance, thereby improving quality of care.

(2) *Eliminating inappropriate care.* A major problem with the U.S. health system is the large amount of health care provided that is entirely unnecessary. Experts have estimated that at least 25% of hospital days, surgeries and medications prescribed are inappropriate.[3] Many people die or are made more sick by such unnecessary medical interventions. Eliminating unnecessary care will not only reduce health care costs, it will also improve quality of care.

It is not easy to eliminate unnecessary care. The NHI should make a major effort to do so in the following ways:

- The more surgeons in an area the more surgeries are performed, and the more hospital beds in an area the more days people spend in the hospital. Controlling the supply of surgeons and hospital beds could help to reduce inappropriate care.
- A new effort—called outcomes research and practice guidelines—has been launched to attempt to reduce inappropriate care. Outcomes research is research designed to show which treatments work and which do not work for particular illnesses. For example, which patients with coronary heart disease should be treated with angioplasty or coronary bypass surgery? Which patients with enlarged prostates should undergo prostate surgery? Based on the results of outcomes research, practice guidelines are being developed to assist physicians and patients to decide which diagnostic tests and which treatments are appropriate for different illnesses.

  By themselves, it is unlikely that outcomes research and practice guidelines will substantially reduce inappropriate care. But together with controls over the supply of high-tech facilities and surgeons and other specialists, outcomes research and practice guidelines may be helpful in reducing inappropriate care and thereby improving quality.
- Studies pioneered by Dr. John Wennberg have shown that similar small geographic areas have widely varying rates of hospitalizations and surgeries. Dr. Wennberg has demonstrated that publicizing this information, especially in areas of high hospitalization and surgery rates, has the effect of reducing surgeries and other care that may be unnecessary.[4] His method may work by embarrassing those physicians responsible for providing excess care. Under national health insurance, it would be easy for the single payer in each state to keep computerized records of different physicians' practice patterns and to investigate physicians who may be performing inappropriate procedures.

(3) *Continuous quality improvement.* A new approach to health care quality has been popularized by Dr. Donald Berwick and others, called continuous quality improvement.[5] The concept is that quality of care can be improved in many cases by analyzing quality of care errors and correcting them through education of health professionals or through improvement of the way the care is organized in a particular hospital or physician office.

Each health care provider and health care institution should be required to establish committees responsible for continuous quality improvement; these committees should be regulated by law and overseen by committees within the health professional organizations and the single payer in each state.

In some cases, poor quality of care is caused by incompetent or impaired health providers; these must be uncovered by the continuous quality improvement committees and barred from the practice of their profession.

What Will Be Done about the Ratio of Specialists to Primary Care Providers?

The United States has far more specialists and fewer primary care providers than we need. Can we truly establish a national health program that is cost effective if there are too many specialists who will always want to perform too many expensive procedures?

This is indeed a major problem and it will take many years or decades to shift the balance of physicians away from specialists and toward primary care providers. But we must start now. First, specialists often earn three to four times what primary care physicians earn; payments to specialists must be drastically reduced such that medical students will be less likely to enter specialty fields. Second, the nation must limit the number of slots available in specialty residencies so that fewer specialists are trained.

Will Health Care Providers Become Available in Inner Cities and Rural Areas?

National health insurance will not automatically fix the maldistribution of medical care in the United States. However, there are some things that single-payer programs in each state can and should do to address this severe problem: (1) provide extra pay to providers who work in underserved areas, (2) train community health workers in underserved areas to provide basic health services with adequate telephone and transportation backup, (3) require physicians and other health professionals to provide a few years of service in underserved areas in return for no-cost medical education.

How Can Costs Be Controlled?

Under the single-payer approach, cost control is simple. Evidence from other nations—Canada and Germany are two examples—proves that when hospitals and doctors are reimbursed by a single-payment mechanism, total health costs can be budgeted and runaway health care inflation can be stopped. If health care inflation is reduced from its present 11% per year to 6%, in the year 2000 our nation will spend $430 billion less on health care than if we continue the current financing system of multiple insurance companies.

Each year the nation would set an overall health budget, and that budget would be apportioned to the single payer in each state according to a formula based on the state's population, health statistics, and other factors. Each state's single payer would set budgets for hospital care, long-term care, physicians' services, etc. Each year, a decision would be made how much to increase the total health budget. Because budgets are fixed, cost control is assured.

Will Rationing Be Needed?

Unlike our current system, a single-payer system has the power to reduce health care costs in three major ways: (1) reduction in administrative costs, which will save from $60 billion to $70 billion each year, (2) reduction in inappropriate care (see the quality of care section above) which may save from $50 billion to $100 billion per year, and (3) reduction in that part of health care inflation that comes from inflated prices for hospital and physician services and from medical supply and pharmaceutical products.

Reducing administrative costs, inappropriate medical care, and excessive price increases will allow our nation to keep health care costs under control without rationing. Cutting costs which do not contribute to good health will prevent us from having to ration needed care that does contribute to good health.

Let us not forget: we spend over 12% of our GNP on health care compared with 9% for Canada; thus the waiting periods that some Canadians experience need not happen in the United States. Our nation has an extremely well-funded health care system. The problem is that 25%–35% of the billions spent on health care is wasted in unnecessary administrative and medical expenditures. If we can reduce the waste, adequate funds are available to provide comprehensive health care to everyone without rationing.

Under a Nationally Budgeted Health System, What Happens If the Money Runs Out?

The money won't run out. Let's take one state and look at its budget in a bit more detail.

- Part of the budget goes for doctors, hospitals, and home care. The single payer and each provider in the state negotiate an annual budget in advance, so the single payer knows exactly how much money will be spent on hospitals and nursing homes before the year even starts.
- Part of the budget goes for HMOs and group practices with salaried physicians. These budgets are also determined in advance, so the single payer can predict how much will be spent on these areas before the year starts.
- Part of the budget goes to fee-for-service physicians. Fees are negotiated between the single payer and the physicians. The difficulty lies in the potential for physicians to provide more and more services, thereby causing the fee-for-service physician budget to be overrun. This is handled by measuring the number of physician services provided every three months, and if the number of services is more than anticipated, physician fees are reduced accordingly. Thus the total amount spent at the end of the year is the amount budgeted.
- Part of the budget goes for pharmaceuticals. As with physicians, if too many prescriptions are ordered, the drug companies are paid less, such that the total amount spent equals the amount budgeted.

These and other methods have been devised in many nations with nationally budgeted health systems to prevent the money running out before the end of the year.

If a Single-Payer System Is Established, What Happens to People Employed by the Insurance Industry and by Hospital Billing Departments?

Many jobs in private insurance companies and hospital billing departments will no longer be needed under a single-payer system. It is extremely important that the people in those jobs be given the opportunity to be trained for alternative employment in the health care sector. Many health care occupations have personnel shortages, for example, nursing, physical and occupational therapy, X-ray and laboratory technology.

When military bases close down, communities can either become ghost towns with high unemployment rates, or they can perform economic conversion planning to switch military employment to civilian jobs. Communities that have done such planning, bringing in new industries, have come through a military base closure without difficulty. The same idea must be utilized for jobs lost through conversion to a single-payer health system: an economic conversion plan to employ those people whose jobs become unnecessary.

Conclusion

As the years go by and health costs stabilize, American families will increasingly feel the benefits of the single-payer approach to national health insurance. Since health insurance would no longer be tied to employment, people would not experience the fear of losing health insurance if they lose their jobs or become sick. People pay through taxes while we are healthy so that we can receive the benefits of the program when we fall sick. The private insurance practice of selling insurance to healthy people and cancelling the coverage or jacking up the premiums when people become sick would be outlawed.

We must realize that a national health insurance program is not a ticket to utopia. It is an attempt to balance the social goals of universal access to health care, and reasonable cost containment.

The basic objectives of national health insurance are simple: to minimize financial barriers to appropriate medical care, to distribute costs fairly, and to contain costs at a reasonable level. Once a structure is in place for meeting these basic concerns we can move on to the complicated questions. Which health care services truly improve the quality of life? What share of our human and material resources should we devote to health care? How shall we reduce the toll now extracted by poverty, ignorance, and addictions? By implementing the single-payer approach to national health insurance, we can turn and face those challenges.

Appendix

Selected articles on the health care service system in the United States and other countries. The articles appeared in the *New England Journal of Medicine,* for 18 months, ending June 30, 1991.

Date	Description	Beginning Page
January 4, 1990	The Increased Needs of Patients in Nursing Homes and Patients Receiving Home Health Care Peter W. Shaughnessy and Andrew M. Kramer	21
January 18, 1990	The Canadian Health Care System: A Canadian Physician's Perspective Adam L. Linton	197
January 25, 1990	U.S. Medical Practice before Medicare and Now—Differences and Consequences Saul S. Radovsky	263
February 8,1990	Reform of the British National Health Service: From White Paper to Bill in Parliament John Lister	410
February 15, 1990	Criteria and Guidelines for Reforming the U.S. Health Care System Stephen M. Shortell and Walter J. McNerney	463
February 15, 1990	Universal Entitlement to Health Care: Can We Get There from Here? David M. Kinzer	467
February 22, 1990	The Doctor-Nurse Game Revisited L. I. Stein, D. T. Watts, and T. Howell	546
March 1, 1990	Occupational Medicine (First of Two Parts) M. R. Cullen, M. G. Cherniack, and L. Rosenstock	594
March 8, 1990	Occupational Medicine (Second of Two Parts) Mark R. Cullen, Martin G. Cherniack, and L. Rosenstock	675

These articles do not include many technical studies of the AIDS epidemic.

References

Preface

1. Morton Levy, *Accounting Goes Public* (Philadelphia: University of Pennsylvania Press, 1977), p. 25.
2. *Health Management Quarterly*, First Quarterly 1989, the Baxter Foundation, p. 5.

Introduction

1. A. Enthoven and R. Kronick, A consumer-choice plan for the 1990s, *New England Journal of Medicine* 320 (1989): 29–37.
2. T. Bodenheimer, Private insurance reform in the 1990s: Can it solve the health care crisis? *International Journal of Health Services* 22 (1991): 197–215.
3. *How California Wastes at Least $10 Billion in Health Care Dollars Each Year* (San Francisco: Health Access, 1991).
4. S. Woolhandler and D. U. Himmelstein, The deteriorating administrative efficiency of the U.S. health care system, *New England Journal of Medicine* 324 (1991) 1,253–58.
5. R. H. Brook, Practice guidelines and practicing medicine, *Journal of the American Medical Association* 262 (1989): 3,027–30.
6. K. R. Levit, M. S. Freeland, and D. R. Waldo, National health care spending trends, 1988, *Health Affairs* 9(2) (1990): 171–84.
7. J. C. Cantor. Expanding health insurance coverage: Who will pay? *Journal of Health Politics, Policy and Law* 15 (1990): 755–78.
8. R. H. Brook, Practice guidelines and practicing medicine, *Journal of the American Medical Association* 262 (1989): 3,027–30.
9. R. H. Brook, Practice guidelines and practicing medicine, *Journal of the American Medical Association* 262 (1989): 3,027–30.

10. J. C. Cantor. Expanding health insurance coverage: Who will pay? *Journal of Health Politics, Policy and Law* 15 (1990): 755–78.

11. R. H. Brook and K. N. Lohr, Will we need to ration effective health care? *Issues in Science and Technology* 3(1) (1986): 68–77.

Chapter 1: The Hill-Burton Shell Game

1. *Encyclopaedia Britannica,* Vol. 10, 1975, p. 1,033.
2. Ibid.
3. Report to Chairman, Select Committee on Hospitals' Better Standards Needed for the Exemptions, p. 2.
4. *The World Almanac,* 1990, p. 844, American Hospital Association.
5. Paul Starr, *The Social Transformation of Medicine* (New York: Basic Books, 1982), p. 278.
6. Ibid., pp. 282, 283.
7. *Hill-Burton Project Register*, U.S. Department of Health, Education and Welfare, July 1, 1947–June 30, 1971, and subsequent reports.
8. Clark C. Havighurst, Regulation of health facilities and services by "certificates of need," *Virginia Law Review,* 59: 1,143, 1,158.
9. Title VI of the Public Health Service Act of August 13, 1946, and Section 29/c of the Act.
10. The Hill-Burton Act, 42 C.F.R. 111(f).
11. *AICPA Hospital Audit Guide,* 4th ed., p. 32.
12. The Hill-Burton Act, 42 C.F.R. 111(f).

Chapter 2: County Hospitals—an Endangered Species

1. Elinor Black and Thomas Bodenheimer, *Closing the Doors on the Poor* (Health Policy Advisory Center, 1975), p. 61.
2. *Report on Consolidation of Hospital Services,* Ad Hoc Committee on Consolidation of Hospital Service Appointed by Yolo County Board of Supervisors, February 1976, p. 29.
3. Ibid., full report and County of Yolo Final Budget 1975–1976: Report compiled by the Board of Supervisors, submitted by Edwin W. Meier, County Executive.

4. *Federal Register* 37 (142): July 22, 1972; Interim Regulation.
5. Amounts listed "as estimated" in the *Hill-Burton Project Register*, p. 56.
6. Report to California Hospital Commission, p. 8.
7. Reconstructed from the Ad Hoc Report because the actual figures were not available.
8. Certification to California Health Facilities Commission for the year ended September 30, 1975.
9. *San Francisco Chronicle,* January 30, 1991, p. A16.
10. Ibid.
11. *Hospital Management Corporations, Creeping Proprietarization,* From Report by the Consumer Commission of the Accreditation of Health Services, Inc. V (2) (June 1978).
12. *Hoover's Profiles of Over 500 Major Corporations* (The Reference Press, Inc., 1990), p. 391.
13. Ibid., p. 302.
14. Visit by API to VMC, February 24, 1977.
15. Visit by API to Merced, February 24, 1977.
16. Exhibit No. 5 of Hyatt's bid proposal and API visit to SNH, June 17, 1977.
17. *The Social Transformation of American Medicine* (New York: Basic Books, 1982), p. 428.

Chapter 3: Nursing Homes—San Francisco and Berkeley, California

1. U.S. Department of Health and Human Services.
2. Peter Kemper, Ph.D., and Christopher M. Murtaugh, Ph.D., Lifetime use of nursing home care, *New England Journal of Medicine* (February 1991): p. 595.
3. API Report, *Financial Study of Skilled Nursing Facilities in San Francisco, 1974–1976,* November 1977, p. 1.
4. California Health Facilities Commission, Sacramento, CA.
5. *Individual Long-Term Care Facility Data for California, Fiscal Years ending December 31, 1979–December 30, 1980,* Report No. 81–14, December 31, 1981.
6. Alta Bates, "Special Report to Friends of Alta Bates Hospital."

Chapter 4: In-Home Services

1. *Homemaker/Home Health Aide Services in the United States,* U.S. Department of HEW, June 1973, pp. 7–10.
2. *Proceedings of the International Congress on Home Health Services,* U.S. Department of HEW, W.A. Publication No. 17, September, 1965.
3. Frank E. Moss and Val J. Halamandaris, *Too Old, Too Sick, Too Bad* (Aspen Systems Corporation, 1977), p. 136.
4. Evelyn Baulch, *Home Care* (Celestial Arts, 1980), pp. 215-23.
5. Janet Zhun Nassif, *The Home Health Care Solution* (New York: Harper & Row, 1985), p. 267.
6. GAO report to the Subcommittee on Health, Committee on Ways and Means, House of Representatives, HRD-89-111, September 1989, p. 10.
7. *Homemaker/Home Health Aide Services in the United States,* U.S. Department of HEW, June 1973, pp. 19–46.
8. Code of Federal Regulations, revised October 1, 1986, 418.204(c), p. 500.
9. Department of Health and Human Services, quoted in *1991 Information Please Almanac,* p. 817.
10. Subcommittee on Health, Committee on Ways and Means, House of Representatives, September 1989, p. 3.

Chapter 5: AIDS

1. Randy Shilts, *And the Band Played On* (New York: St. Martin's Press, 1987), p. 37.
2. U.S. Department of Health and Human Services HIV/AIDS Surveillance, March 1989, p. 5.
3. *The New York Times Magazine,* April 19, 1987, p. 33.
4. Louise L. Hay, *The AIDS Book* (Santa Monica: The Hay House, 1988), p. 2.
5. Victor Gong, M.D., and Norman Rudnick, editors, *AIDS Facts and Issues* (New Brunswick: Rutgers University Press, 1987), p. 121.
6. *The Random House Encyclopedia,* 1990, p. 2,281.
7. Victor Gong, M.D., and Norman Rudnick, editors, *AIDS Facts

and Issues (New Brunswick: Rutgers University Press, 1987), p. 140.

8. Randy Shilts, *And the Band Played On* (New York: St. Martin's Press, 1987), p. 186.
9. *San Francisco Chronicle,* March 5, 1987.
10. Bruce Nussbaum, *Good Intentions* (New York: The Atlantic Monthly Press, 1990), p. 16.
11. Ibid., p. 13.
12. Ibid., p. 15.
13. *San Francisco Chronicle,* March 22, 1991.
14. Bruce Nussbaum, *Good Intentions* (New York: The Atlantic Monthly Press, 1990), p. 4.
15. Sandra Panem, *AIDS Bureaucracy* (Cambridge: Harvard University Press, 1988), p. 83.

Chapter 6: Alternative Health Care Financing

1. Paul Starr, *The Social Transformation of American Medicine* (New York: Basic Books, 1982), p. 272.
2. Robert J. Myers, Medicare, McCanan Foundation, 1970, p. 20.
3. *San Francisco Chronicle,* December 16, 1983.
4. David A. Swope, *The Wall Street Journal,* January 3, 1984.
5. A Three-Year Study by Alfred J. Kahn and Sheila B. Kamerman of Columbia's School of Social Work, Financed by the Social Security Administration.
6. Quoted by the *San Francisco Chronicle,* January 26, 1984.
7. Sylvia A. Law, *Blue Cross: What Went Wrong?* (Cambridge: Harvard University Press, 1974), pp. 39–41.
8. U.S. Department of Health and Human Services, *HCFA 83-02153* (pamphlet).
9. *The World Almanac,* 1990, Table of Consumer Price Indexes for Selected Groups, p. 88.
10. *The New York Times,* June 18, 1991.
11. *The World Almanac,* 1990, p. 5.
12. Richard Severo and Lewis Milford, *The Wages of War* (New York: Simon & Schuster, 1981), p. 61.
13. *The Random House Encyclopedia,* 1990, p. 2,617.
14. Ibid., p. 65.
15. Richard Severo and Lewis Milford, *The Wages of War* (New York: Simon & Schuster, 1981), p. 129.
16. Ibid., p. 138.

17. Paul Starr, *The Discarded Army* (Charterhouse, 1973), p. 76.

18. Harrison E. Salisbury, ed., *Vietnam Reconsidered* (New York: Harper & Row, 1984), p. 185.

19. Ibid., pp. 193–95.

20. Department of Veterans Affairs, Annual Report, 1988, p. 224.

21. *The Patient is Critical,* the American Legion, January 1990, pp. 38–39.

22. Harrison E. Salisbury, ed., *Vietnam Reconsidered* (New York: Harper Row, 1984), p. 198.

23. *The American Legion Magazine,* the American Legion, September 1989, p. 41.

24. Jill Bloom, *HMO* (Los Angeles: The Body Press, 1987).

25. *Facts, 1990,* Kaiser Permanente, pp. 1–6.

26. *San Francisco Chronicle,* May 8, 1991, p. 1.

27. Blue Shield of California, July 1990.

Chapter 7: Mental Health Services and the Homeless

1. Richard J. Wagner, M.D., F.A.C.P, *Medical and Health Encyclopedia* (J. G. Ferguson Publishing Company, 1986), pp. 532–35.

2. E. Fuller Torrey, M.D., *Nowhere to Go* (New York: Harper & Row, 1988), p. 57.

3. Dr. Parran's opening statement before congressional hearings to form a National Neuropsychiatric Institute.

4. Paul Starr, *The Social Transformation of American Medicine* (New York: Basic Books, 1982), pp. 342–47.

5. *Patients in Mental Institutions,* Rockville, MD: National Institute of Mental Health, 1955.

6. Ibid., 1984.

7. E. Fuller Torrey, M.D., *Nowhere to Go* (New York: Harper & Row, 1988), pp. 34–35.

8. *Down and Out in America* (Chicago: University of Chicago Press, 1989), p. 146.

Chapter 8: Waste, Fraud, and Abuse

1. Steffie Woolhandler, M.D., M.P.H., and David V. Himmelstein, M.D., *New England Journal of Medicine* (May 2, 1991): pp. 1,253–58.

2. *Staff Report on Fraud and Abuse Among Practitioners Participating in the Medicaid Program,* Washington, D.C.: U.S. Government Printing Office, 1976, p. 7.
3. Frank E. Moss and Val J. Halamandaris, *Too Old, Too Sick, Too Bad* (Aspen Publishers, Inc.), p. 74.
4. Ibid., p. 173.
5. Ibid., p. 34.
6. Paul Starr, *The Social Transformation of American Medicine* (New York: Basic Books, 1982), p. 295.
7. *Report by the Select Committee on Aging—House of Representatives,* Washington, D.C.: U.S. Government Printing Office, 1981.
8. Harvard Medical Practice Study Group, "Patients, Doctors and Lawyers: Medical Injury, Malpractice Litigation and Patient Compensation in New York," 1990.

Chapter 9: Preventive Medicine

1. As reported in *JAMA,* July 21, 1989, 262: 376–79.
2. *JAMA,* July 21, 1989, 262: 376–79.
3. *JAMA,* July 21, 1989, 262: 376 79.
4. *U.S. National Center for Health Statistics, Vital Statistics of the United States, Annual* (Table 110).
5. Reported in the *San Francisco Chronicle,* February 7, 1991, p. A6.
6. Etienne-Emile Baulieu with Mort Rosenblum, *The "Abortion Pill,"* (New York: Simon & Schuster, 1991), p. 15.
7. *Health United States and Prevention Profile,* Washington, D.C.: U.S. Government Printing Office, 1983, p. 260.
8. *Health United States,* Washington, D.C.: U.S. Government Printing Office, 1990, p. 91.
9. *The Random House Encyclopedia,* 1990, p. 2,548.
10. Kathleen Whalen Fitzgerald, Ph.D., *Alcoholism, the Genetic Inheritance* (New York: Doubleday, 1988), p. vii.
11. *The Diagnostic and Statistical Manual: The Diagnostic and Statistical Manual of Mental Disorders, DSM-III,* the American Psychiatric Association, 1980, p. 129.
12. Ibid., pp. 130–31.
13. Kathleen Whalen Fitzgerald, Ph.D., *Alcoholism, the Genetic Inheritance* (New York: Doubleday, 1988), p. 213.
14. *Encyclopaedia Britannica,* 1982, Vol. 5, p. 1,041.

15. *DSM-III*, the American Psychiatric Association, 1980, pp. 163–68.
16. *U.S. News and World Report,* August 10, 1991, p. 51.
17. *OSAP Prevention Monograph-2, Prevention of Mental Disorders, Alcohol and Other Drug Use in Children and Adolescents,* U.S. Department of Health and Human Services, 1989.
18. *Hazard Elimination Procedures for Leaded Paints in Housing,* U.S. Department of Commerce, May 1973, p. 1 et alii.
19. *San Francisco Chronicle,* August 15, 1991, p. A4.

Conclusion: The Single-Payer Approach to National Health Insurance by Thomas S. Bodenheimer, M.D.

1. S. Woolhandler and D. U. Himmelstein, The deteriorating administrative efficiency of the U.S. health care system, *New England Journal of Medicine* 324 (1991): 1,253–58.
2. Canadian Health Insurance: Lessons for the United States, Washington, D.C.: U.S. General Accounting Office, 1991.
3. R. H. Brook, and K. N. Lohr, Will we need to ration effective health care! *Issues in Science and Technology* 3(1) (1986): 68–77.
4. *Perspectives on Quality in American Health Care* (New York: McGraw-Hill Book Co., 1988).
5. D. M. Berwick, A. B. Godfrey, and J. Roessner, *Curing Health Care* (San Francisco: Jossey-Bass Publishers, 1990).

Index